Arthroscopy
of the
Wrist and Elbow

Arthroscopy
of the
Wrist and Elbow

Gary G. Poehling, M.D.
Professor and Chairman
Department of Orthopaedic Surgery
The Bowman Gray School of Medicine
Wake Forest University
Winston-Salem, North Carolina

ASSOCIATE EDITORS

L. Andrew Koman, M.D.
Professor
Department of Orthopaedic Surgery
The Bowman Gray School of Medicine
Wake Forest University
Winston-Salem, North Carolina

Thomas L. Pope, Jr., M.D.
Professor
Department of Radiology
The Bowman Gray School of Medicine
Wake Forest University
Winston-Salem, North Carolina

David B. Siegel, M.D.
Catalina Orthopaedic Surgery
Tucson, Arizona

RAVEN PRESS   NEW YORK

Raven Press, Ltd., 1185 Avenue of the Americas, New York, New York 10036

Printed and bound in Singapore

Library of Congress Cataloging-in-Publication Data

Arthroscopy of the wrist and elbow / editor-in chief, Gary G. Poehling;
   associate editors, L. Andrew Koman, Thomas L. Pope, Jr., David B. Siegel.
      p. cm.
    Includes bibliographical references and index.
    ISBN 0-7817-0194-5
    1. Wrist—Endoscopic surgery.   2. Elbow—Endoscopic surgery.
   3. Wrist—Examination.   4. Elbow—Examination.   5. Arthroscopy.
   I. Poehling, Gary.
    [DNLM: 1. Arthroscopy—methods. 2. Wrist—surgery. 3. Elbow—
   surgery. WE 830 A787 1994]
   RD559.A77 1994
   617.5'74059—dc20
   DNLM/DLC
   for Library of Congress   93-42821

9 8 7 6 5 4 3 2 1

This work was made possible by three important people in my life.
My wife, Sandra (Sandy) Poehling,
and my parents, Gerhard G. and Anne E. Poehling,
a heartfelt thanks for your continued support and encouragement.
G.G.P.

To my wife, Leigh,
my children, Amy and Alex,
and the memories of my mother, Carolyn Koman,
and my father-in-law, Don Emerson.
L.A.K.

To the people who put up with me on a day to day basis,
my wife, Lou,
and my sons, David and Jason.
For the support of my mother, Florence,
and my brother, Robin.
And, especially, to the memory of my father,
Thomas L. Pope, Sr.,
one of the finest role models a son could ever have.
T.L.P., Jr.

To Linda, Molly, Emma, and Abby,
for making my life great.
And to the orthopaedic residents at
Bowman Gray School of Medicine
who were a pleasure to teach.
D.B.S.

———

Contents

Contributors

James R. Andrews, M.D.
Clinical Professor, Department of Orthopaedics and Sports Medicine, University of Virginia Medical School, Charlottesville, Virginia; Alabama Sports Medicine and Orthopaedic Center, Suite 200, 1201 11th Avenue, South Birmingham, Alabama 35205

William H. Bowers, M.D.
Associate Clinical Professor of Hand Surgery, Department of Surgery, Medical College of Virginia, Richmond, Virginia; Hand Surgery Specialists, Ltd., 7650 East Parham Road, Richmond, Virginia 23294

William G. Carson, Jr., M.D.
Assistant Clinical Professor, Department of Orthopaedic Surgery, University of South Florida, Tampa, Florida; The Sports Medicine Clinic of Tampa, 3006 West Azeele Street, Tampa, Florida 33609

Stephen J. Chabon, P.A.-C.
Department of Orthopaedic Surgery, The Bowman Gray School of Medicine, Wake Forest University Medical Center, Medical Center Boulevard, Winston-Salem, North Carolina 27157-1070; current address: *The Hand Center of Greensboro, Greensboro, North Carolina 27401*

Michael Y. M. Chen, M.D.
Associate Professor, Department of Radiology, The Bowman Gray School of Medicine, Wake Forest University, Medical Center Boulevard, Winston-Salem, North Carolina 27157-1088

William P. Cooney, M.D.
Professor, Department of Orthopedic Surgery, Mayo Medical School and Mayo Clinic, 200 First Street, SW, Rochester, Minnesota 55905

Judy L. Cooper, R.N.
Clinical Orthopaedic Nurse Specialist, Tuckahoe Orthopaedic Associates, Ltd., 8919 Three Chopt Road, Richmond, Virginia 23229

Evan F. Ekman, M.D.
Department of Orthopaedic Surgery, The Bowman Gray School of Medicine, Wake Forest University, Medical Center Boulevard, Winston-Salem, North Carolina 27157-1070

Donald C. Ferlic, M.D.
Associate Clinical Professor, Department of Orthopedic Surgery, University of Colorado Health Sciences Center, Suite 5000, 1601 East 19th Street, Denver, Colorado 80205

L. Andrew Koman, M.D.
Professor, Department of Orthopaedic Surgery, The Bowman Gray School of Medicine, Wake Forest University, Medical Center Boulevard, Winston-Salem, North Carolina 27157-1070

David M. Lichtman, M.D.
Rear Admiral, Medical Corps, USN; Commander, National Naval Medical Center, Bethesda, Maryland; Professor and Head, Division of Orthopaedic Surgery, Uniformed Services University of the Health Sciences, Bethesda, Maryland 20889

Patrick J. McKenzie, M.D.
Orthopaedic Associates of Green Bay, 704 S. Webster, Green Bay, Wisconsin 54301

John F. Meyers, M.D.
Associate Clinical Professor, Medical College of Virginia, Richmond, Virginia; Tuckahoe Orthopaedic Associates, Ltd., 8919 Three Chopt Road, Richmond, Virginia 23229

Andrew K. Palmer, M.D.
Professor, Department of Orthopedic Surgery, Director of Hand Surgery, State University of New York at Syracuse, East Adams Street, Syracuse, New York 13202

Gary G. Poehling, M.D.
Professor and Chairman, Department of Orthopaedic Surgery, The Bowman Gray School of Medicine, Wake Forest University, Medical Center Boulevard, Winston-Salem, North Carolina 27157-1070

Thomas L. Pope, Jr., M.D.
Professor, Department of Radiology, The Bowman Gray School of Medicine, Wake Forest University, Medical Center Boulevard, Winston-Salem, North Carolina 27157-1088

James H. Roth, M.D.
Professor, Department of Surgery, Division of Orthopaedics, University of Western Ontario; Director, Hand and Upper Limb Center, St. Joseph's Health Center, 268 Grosvenor Street, London, Ontario, N6A 4LG, Canada

David S. Ruch, M.D.
Assistant Professor, Department of Orthopaedic Surgery, The Bowman Gray School of Medicine, Wake Forest University, Medical Center Boulevard, Winston-Salem, North Carolina; and 251 Lochridge Drive, Durham, North Carolina 27713

David B. Siegel, M.D.
Catalina Orthopaedic Surgery, 2424 North Wyatt Drive, Tucson, Arizona 85712-3125

Terry L. Whipple, M.D.
Clinical Professor, Department of Orthopaedic Surgery, The Bowman Gray School of Medicine, Wake Forest University, Winston-Salem, North Carolina; Department of Orthopaedic Surgery, University of Virginia, Charlottesville, Virginia; Tuckahoe Orthopaedic Associates Ltd., 8919 Three Chopt Road, Richmond, Virginia 23229

Preface

Over the past decade, interest in the wrist and elbow has escalated. We have learned a great deal about these joints through application of new technologies such as arthroscopy and radiology. Historically, the early development of wrist arthroscopy began in May of 1985 in Salzburg, Austria, during a meeting of the International Society of the Knee. Terry L. Whipple, James H. Roth (two colleagues who were trained at Duke), and I decided to meet over dinner to discuss old times. Instead of talking about old times, we quickly discovered that each had done preliminary wrist cadaver work using arthroscopy. Terry Whipple and Jim Roth had already done some clinical cases, so we shared our findings. We needed to learn more, and the strategy we chose was to involve many others in the development of wrist arthroscopy. It was clear that to be able to apply the arthroscopic technique to wrist disorders we required more knowledge about the wrist.

In order to tweak the interest of wrist experts, Jim Roth prepared an article and an instructional course in wrist arthroscopy. Terry Whipple developed a teaching model that could be used in a course that I was to organize with Drs. Whipple and Roth and on the advice of three colleagues, L. Andrew Koman, Jim Urbaniak, and William H. Bowers. Leading experts in wrist surgery were invited to our meeting held at Graylyn Estates of Wake Forest University in Winston-Salem, North Carolina, in January of 1986. The enthusiasm and energy at the meeting oftentimes made it hard to tell who was putting on the meeting and who was attending. From that meeting sprang much understanding from all points of view with regard to wrist abnormalities.

This book illustrates progress of wrist and elbow arthroscopy since that meeting in January of 1986. We hope to rekindle the enthusiasm for continued advancement of treatment algorithms that are safe, effective, and economical, and that return quality function to patients with upper extremity impairment.

There are many surgeons who have a primary interest in upper extremity treatment. This book provides a comprehensive presentation of minimally invasive techniques applied to their field of interest.

Gary G. Poehling, M.D.

WRIST

Arthroscopy of the Wrist

Introduction and Indications

Terry L. *Whipple*, M.D.

The development of techniques for arthroscopic examination of various joints has provided a world of new understanding of anatomy, mechanics, and pathology in orthopedics. The wrist is a complex system of articulations that now has been subjected to arthroscopic exploration with greater than anticipated success and revelation. Although attempted sporadically from time to time in various centers, primarily in Japan and the United States, it was not until 1986 that wrist arthroscopy began to gain widespread acceptance. The techniques developed and reported by Whipple et al. in the *Journal of Arthroscopy and Related Surgery* proved successful for other clinicians as well, and the prevalence of wrist pain with normal radiographic findings has prompted a surprising enthusiasm for arthroscopic examination of the wrist (1).

The following chapters on wrist arthroscopy will address why, when, and how to employ arthroscopic techniques to the wrist. Specific pathologic conditions amenable to arthroscopic evaluation or treatment will be discussed in detail. To date, the orthopedic literature contains little information about wrist arthroscopy, so references are scant, unfortunately.

Wrist arthroscopy has emerged as a natural evolutionary development from the successful applications of arthroscopic techniques in other joints. Soft tissue pathology within or around joints is especially troublesome to define or quantify without the advantage of direct examination. Numerous radiolucent structures of the wrist cause pain or dysfunction but elude diagnosis by conventional imaging techniques and experienced physical examination. Intercarpal ligament tears or perforations of the triangular fibrocartilage may be revealed by arthrography, but there is a significant incidence of false-negative arthrograms. Articular cartilage is virtually impossible to evaluate in the wrist before secondary osseous changes develop.

Technological improvements in the manufacture of optical devices have allowed the development of miniature arthroscopes with angled lenses and large, clear fields of view. The scopes can be manipulated safely between the fragile articular surfaces of the wrist to allow direct inspection of the intraarticular anatomy. More sensitive, lighter weight video cameras further enlarge the visual image from these arthroscopes with impressive color and resolution and reduce the strain on both surgeon and equipment. Considering then the substantial morbidity of wrist arthrotomy, minimally invasive arthroscopic techniques for the wrist have tremendous appeal. When internal structures can be thoroughly examined and manipulated with little surgical trauma and greatly reduced scarring and recuperation (which would result from conventional wrist arthrotomy), so much the better for the patient. In addition, with greatly improved illumination and magnification, the examination becomes all the more thorough.

Indications for wrist arthroscopy may occur when the diagnosis is confirmed, equivocal, or unresolved. With the confirmed diagnosis, such as arthrographically proven perforations of the triangular fibrocartilage, arthroscopy can help to define the size and precise location of the lesion and thereby facilitate planning of surgical approach and definitive treatment. Associated soft tissue lesions such as articular cartilage defects may also be discovered or ruled out arthroscopically.

When preoperative evaluation of the wrist leaves the primary diagnosis uncertain, arthroscopic examination may provide clarifying information. For example, ulnar wrist pain associated with chronic rotatory scapholunate dissociation remains a diagnostic enigma, even if the technetium bone scan is positive on both sides of the joint. An associated articular defect on the proximal pole of hamate would best be revealed by arthroscopic examination.

Should diagnosis remain obscure despite an otherwise thorough evaluation, arthroscopic examination of the wrist will provide useful information without compounding the situation by surgical intervention. If, for example, disabling symptoms persist following reasonable conservative treatment in a compensable injury and if there remains no objective evidence of pathology, direct visual examination may provide the most reliable diagnostic coup de grace.

In addition, since the development of appropriately sized instruments designed specifically for use in small joints under arthroscopic control, many wrist lesions can be successfully treated with the added advantage of minimally invasive techniques. Surgical exposure of the wrist is too often associated with residual stiffness or dystrophy. Reduction of surgical trauma, if the definitive treatment can be accomplished as well with less invasive measures, is always of functional and economic advantage.

REFERENCE

1. Whipple TL, Marotta JJ, Powell JH. Techniques of wrist arthroscopy. *Arthroscopy* 1986;244–252.

Arthroscopic Anatomy of the Wrist

William H. Bowers, M.D., and Terry L. Whipple, M.D.

Presentation of the anatomy of the wrist for a book on arthroscopy creates special circumstances. Great advances have only recently occurred in the gross anatomic study of wrist articulation. This 10-bone, 15- to 20-ligament complex is slowly giving up its secrets to motivated anatomists and surgeons, who use classic techniques of dissection, newer techniques of imaging, and biomechanical research. The technique of arthroscopy has pushed the frontier ahead by a large measure, allowing us a magnified look at the joint from within and in a specimen (the patient) that provides us with normal colors and textures. To place this technique in its proper perspective as a research tool and at the same time as an interventionist modality is difficult.

The anatomy, seen living and from within, is awesome. To alter it without understanding its biomechanics and classic anatomy is not recommended. The recent volumes on the wrist by Taleisnik (5) and Lichtman (3) and the wrist and distal radioulnar joint chapters in Green's *Operative Hand Surgery* by Green (2), Bowers (1), and Palmer (4) are strongly recommended to the reader. With these thoughts firmly in mind there are questions of anatomy a surgeon employing the technique of arthroscopy should ask himself.

1. What portal of entry should I choose to see the structure of my interest?
2. How can I find this portal using known topographic anatomic landmarks?
3. What superficial anatomic structures of importance are in the immediate vicinity of this portal?
4. How can I avoid injuring these structures if I choose this portal?
5. How do I enter this portal?
6. What will I see upon entering this portal?
7. What are the intraarticular anatomic structures in the immediate vicinity of my initial entry field of view?
8. What can I *not* see well with this portal?
9. What is this portal's best use?

This chapter, on anatomy, will deal with questions 1–3 and 5–8. Questions 4 and 9 will be dealt with more fully in other chapters. The location of the designated portals can be found by the diagrams shown in Figs. 1 and 2 and a review of the location of known palpable landmarks on one's own wrist. The palpation of tendon borders requires active tension within the neuromusculotendinous unit. Locate these landmarks before anesthesia if possible. Landmarks to be located are listed in Table 1 along with the portals requiring their review. The letters in Table 1 correspond with the locations shown by letter in Figs. 1 and 2.

ARTHROSCOPIC ANATOMY OF PORTAL 1–2

To find portal 1–2 find *proximally* the distal margin of the radius at the radiocarpal joint. Find *dorsally* the extensor pollicis longus (EPL) (D in Figs. 1 and 2) and *volarly* the abductor pollicis longus, extensor pollicis brevis bundle (C in Figs. 1 and 2). Crossing this trapezoidal window is the radial artery (B in Figs. 1 and 2). Find this by palpation or Doppler. Avoid by staying proximally and dorsally in the window for your puncture. The radial sensory nerve (shown overlying tendons) is variable and occasionally palpable. Avoid by proper skin incision. For

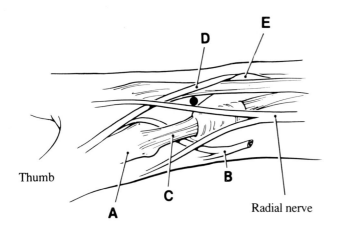

FIG. 1. Radial side of the right wrist with hand to the left. The location of the radial sensory nerve is variable, but a common arrangement is depicted. The heavy black line outlines the trapezoidal area within which one will find portal 1–2. A, base of thumb metacarpal; B, radial artery; C, first dorsal compartment tendons as they bridge the radial styloid–metacarpal interval; D, extensor pollicis longus; E, Lister's tubercle.

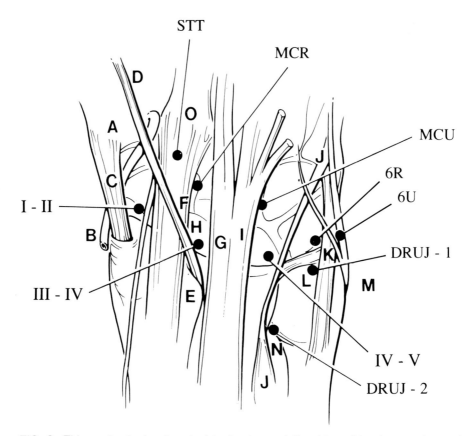

FIG. 2. This anatomic drawing depicts the true relationships of tendons and carpal bones as they rest in a slightly distracted wrist as one might see at arthroscopy. The overlap between radius and proximal carpal row cannot be ignored, as most of the proximal one-half of the scaphoid and lunate lie under the dorsal margin of the radius. A, thumb metacarpal base; B, radial artery; C, first dorsal compartment tendons; D, extensor pollicis longus tendon; E, Lister's tubercle; F, ulnar border of common wrist extensor tendons at waist of scaphoid; G, radial border of common finger extensor tendons at radial margin; H, proximal articular surface of the scaphoid; I, ulnar border of common finger extensor tendons over lunate; J, extensor digiti minimi tendon; K, extensor carpi ulnaris; L, ulnar articular dome; M, ulnar styloid; N, axilla between radius and ulna at radioulnar joint; O, base of index and long metacarpals (carpal boss). The portals are as follows: STT, scaphotrapeziotrapezoid; MCR, midcarpal radial; MCU, midcarpal ulnar; 6R, 6 radial; 6U, 6 ulnar; DRUJ-1 and DRUJ-2, distal radioulnar joint 1 and 2.

TABLE 1. *Entry portals for wrist arthroscopy*

Portal and anatomic landmark	
Portal 1–2 A. Base of thumb metacarpal B. Radial artery C. Abductor pollicis longus, extensor pollicis brevis tendon bundle between radial styloid and base of thumb metacarpal D. Extensor pollicis longus	*Portal 6R and 6U* K. Extensor carpi ulnaris L. Prominent ulnar articular surface (forearm neutral or pronated) M. Ulnar styloid N. Radioulnar axilla just proximal to radioulnar articulation
Portal 3–4 D. Extensor pollicis longus E. Lister's tubercle F. Ulnar edge of ECRL at radiocarpal joint G. Radial edge of common extensors at radiocarpal joint H. Prominence of scaphoid's radial articular face (wrist volar flexed)	*Radial midcarpal portal* O. Carpometacarpal joint between the index and long metacarpals and the trapezoid–capitate joint (carpal boss) *Ulnar midcarpal portal* P. Fourth metacarpal midshaft axis Q. Four-corner intersection of the capitate, lunate, triquetrum, and hemate
Portal 4–5 I. Ulnar edge of common extensors at radiocarpal joint J. Extensor digiti minimi at radiocarpal joint (move the little finger independently and palpate for motion of this tendon at radiocarpal joint)	*STT portal* R. Second metacarpal midshaft axis S. Extensor pollicis longus tendon T. Scaphotrapeziotrapezoid articulation

the arthroscopic anatomy of portal 1–2 refer to Figs. 3–5. Your field of view will include radially the radioscaphocapitate (RSC) ligament as it originates from the volar margin of the radial styloid, passes volar to the waist of the scaphoid, and ends on the volar body of the capitate. The division between this radialmost ligament and the adjacent ligaments [the combined radiolunotriquetral ligament (RLT) and radiolunate (RL) ligament] is very distinct (see arrow 1 in Fig. 3). The RL ligament is somewhat obscured by a very prominent tuft of synovium and ligament-like tissue that seemingly connects the radius, lunate, and scapholunate interosseous ligament (SLL). This tuft of tissue (arrow 2 in Fig. 3) is easily found on inspection through portals 1–2, 3–4, and 4–5. It is the "ligament of Kuenz and Testut" or radioscapholunate (RSL). This landmark orients you to the SLL distally, the articular surface of the scaphoid to its distal left, the articular surface of the lunate to its distal right, the scaphoid fossa of the radius (proximal left), and the lunate fossa of the radius (proximal right). The proximal ridge dividing these two fossae can easily be seen with this portal. Further to the right the margin between the radius and triangular fibrocartilage (TFC) can be seen (arrow 3 in Fig. 3) but appreciated more by a distinct difference in texture, the radial cartilage relatively firm, the TFC relatively soft. The arthroscopic penetration through portal 1–2 will produce a progression of views of these structures (Fig. 4A–C) as you go from radial to ulnar within the joint. The general view for portals 1–2 is shown in the area in Fig. 3 between the proximal carpal bones and the radius. Structures not well seen with this entry portal are those of the extreme ulnar half of the joint and the structures under and radial to the penetration (radial styloid tip, dorsal rim of radial styloid).

ARTHROSCOPIC ANATOMY OF PORTAL 3–4

The portal is found by locating the wrist dimple 1 cm distal to Lister's tubercle (E in Fig. 2, A in Fig. 5). Palpate the distal edge of the radius between the ulnar border of the extensor carpi radialus longus (ECRL) (F in Fig. 2) and radial margin of the common extensors (G in Fig. 2), flex the wrist, and feel the articular surface of the scaphoid emerge from the scaphoid fossa of the radius (H in Fig. 2). Enter here with the scope directed 10° proximally. Your entry will be directly over the ridge dividing the scaphoid and lunate fossa and directly ahead of you will be the synovial tuft of the ligament of Testut (arrow 2 in Fig. 3, Figs. 6 and 7). You will be centered on field of view B in Fig. 4 *and* as shown in Fig. 8. Moving the *hand* holding the scope ulnarward will bring the radialmost structures seen in Figs. 7 and 8 in view (the radial styloid and the radioscaphocapitate ligament). Moving the hand holding the scope radially will allow a good view of the lunate, the lunotriquetral interosseous ligament (LT), and the TFC.

ARTHROSCOPIC ANATOMY OF PORTAL 4–5

This portal is located between the ulnar margin of the common extensors (I in Fig. 2) and the extensor digiti minimi (J in Fig. 2) at the edge of the radius. It is 1 cm directly ulnarward to the 3–4 portal discussed above. The portal is identified on Fig. 5(b) and on Fig. 9(b), which shows the capsular entry in relationship to portal 6R and the distal radioulnar joint. Entry into this portal is over the dorsal margin of the radius just at its junction with the TFC (compare Figs. 10 and 11). Directly ahead

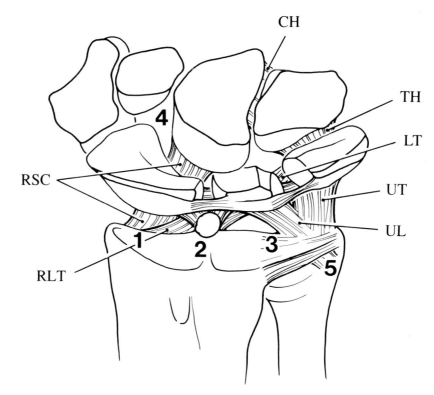

FIG. 3. This exploded view of the wrist shows relatively true carpal anatomic relationships from the dorsum as observed by an arthroscopist. The volar ligaments seen in the depths between the carpal bones can often be seen well, perhaps better than by any other technique. 1, division between radioscaphocapitate ligament (RSC) and combined radiolunotriquetral (RLT) and radiolunate ligaments; 2, synovial tuft covering the ligament of Kuenz and Testut or radioscapholunate ligament; 3, margin of radius and triangular fibrocartilage; 4, scaphocapitate fossa, the portal for the radial midcarpal puncture; 5, portal DRUJ-1. Other labeled structures: UL, ulnolunate ligament; UT, ulnotriquetral ligament; LT (volar), lunotriquetral ligament; TH, triquetrohamate ligament; CH, capitohamate ligament.

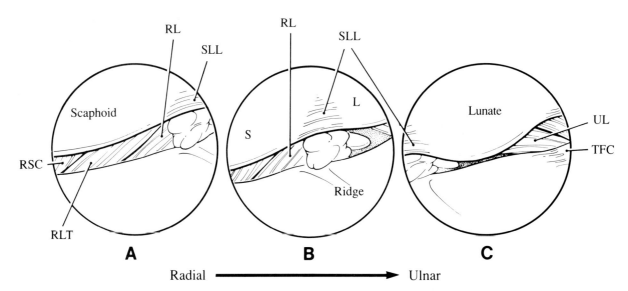

FIG. 4. Sequential drawings of the radial carpal arthroscopic views seen from shallow to deep through portal 1–2. Compare with Figs. 6 and 7. Ligaments: L, lunate; RL, radiolunate; RLT, radiolunotriquetral; RSC, radioscaphocapitate; S, scaphoid; SLL, scapholunate interosseous; TFC, triangular fibrocartilage; UL, ulnolunate.

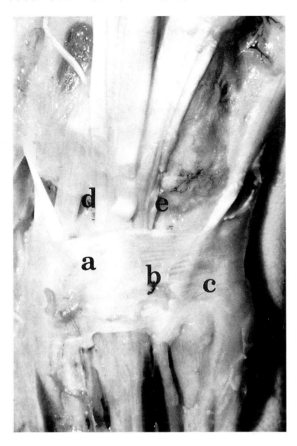

FIG. 5. The dorsal retinaculum and tendon structures of the dorsum of the wrist. This figure should be compared with Fig. 2. Portals marked are: a, 3–4; b, 4–5; c, 6R portal; both radial (d) and ulnar (e) midcarpal portals.

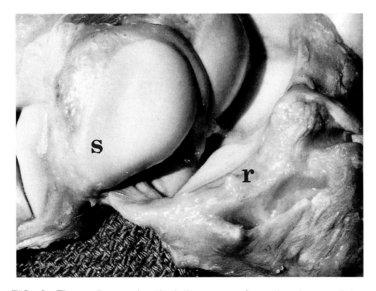

FIG. 6. The radiocarpal articulations seen from the dorsoradial view. The scaphoid (s) is flexed and to the left. The radius (r) is to the right. The orientation provides a gross view of the structures seen from portal 1–2. The most radial volar ligament is the radioscaphocapitate (RSC) and adjacent to it the combined radiolunotriquetral (RLT) and radiolunate (RL) ligaments. A large portion of this ligament complex passes volar to the lunate to insert on the triquetral bone (gaining its designation) while an equally large portion inserts into the lunate. The scapholunate interosseous ligament is seen well as a convex structure between the scaphoid and lunate. In the "live" condition this ligament is on stretch and often cannot be seen nearly as well. In fact, it may appear as a concave interval between the scaphoid and lunate (see Figs. 4 and 8).

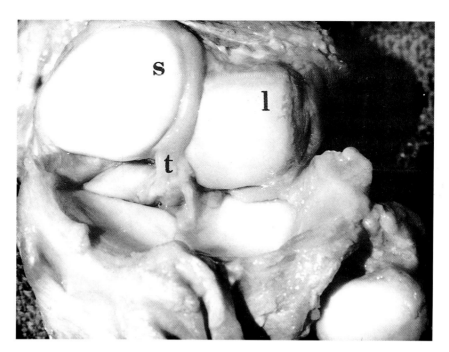

FIG. 7. The radiocarpal articulation seen from a dorsal view. The carpus is flexed and to the top of the picture showing the articular surfaces of proximal scaphoid (s) and the lunate (l). The scapholunate interosseous ligament is convex. The volar ligaments are the RSC (most radial) and the RLT/RL ligament complex (see Fig. 6). The synovial tuft (t) appearing to connect radius and scapholunate ligament is covering the ligament of Kuenz and Testut, or RSL ligament. The articular ridge between the scaphoid and lunate facets on the radius is seen well. The view is a gross representation of the field available through the 3–4 portal.

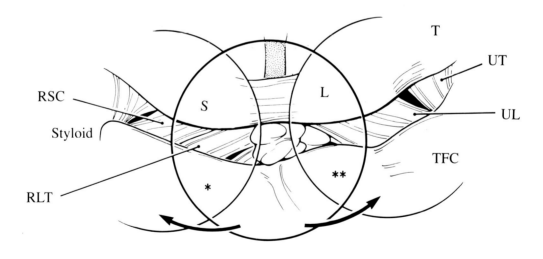

* Scaphoid fossa   **Lunate fossa

FIG. 8. The radiocarpal articulation is seen from portal 3–4. Compare with Fig. 5. The ligament-like structures seen to the extreme left of the radioscaphocapitate (RSC) ligament is the capsule underlying the tendons of the first dorsal compartment. This capsular condensation (often called the radial collateral ligament) is not a true collateral ligament as it lies volar to the flexion extension axis of the wrist. It ends distally on the trapezium. UT, ulnotriquetral ligament. For other abbreviations, see legend to Fig. 4.

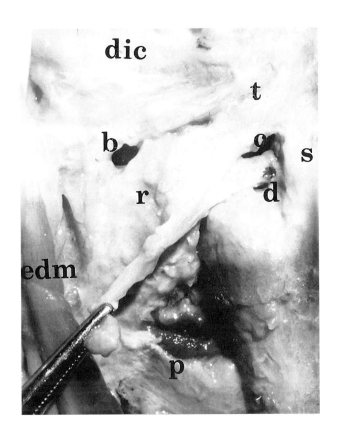

FIG. 9. The dorsal wrist capsule seen from an ulnar orientation. The carpus occupies the top one-half of the photo with the ulnar articular surface and styloid (s) to the right and the radius (r) to the left. The apertures are portals 4–5 (b), 6R (c), and DRUJ-1 (d), the latter two straddling the TFC. The dorsal intercarpal ligament (dic) and proximal and distal dorsal radiotriquetral ligament (b, t and r, t) all converge to the triquetrum (t). The muscles are pronator quadratus (p) and extensor digiti minimi (edm).

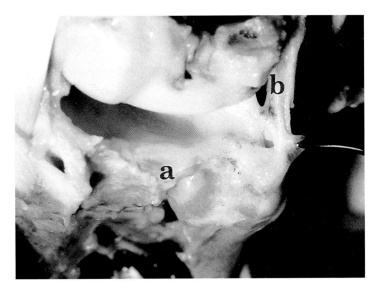

FIG. 10. The ulnocarpal articulation seen grossly as it might appear on 4–5 portal arthroscopy (a). Compare with Fig. 11. The clamp is on the meniscal homologue, which has been dissected free from point a and elevated to show the pisotriquetral recess (b) and the prestyloid recess just proximal. Note the smooth and distinct continuation from the lunate fossa cartilage covering the radius to the TFC. The two carpal bones seen are lunate (left) and triquetrum (right). The ulnar articular dome can be seen emerging from under the TFC.

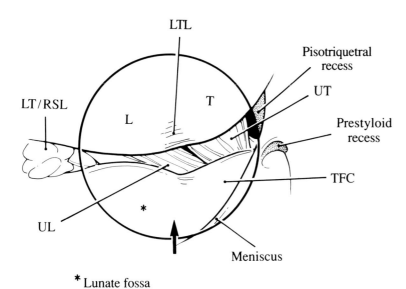

FIG. 11. Arthroscopic view through portal 4–5. The meniscal homologue (see Fig. 10) may be seen to the lower right. This meniscal structure, often overlying the TFC (occasionally fused to it), covers the entry to the prestyloid recess. UL, ulnolunate ligament; UT, ulnotriquetral ligament; LTL, lunotriquetral interosseous ligament; LT/RSL, ligament of Testut, radioscapholunate ligament; L, lunate; T, triquetrum.

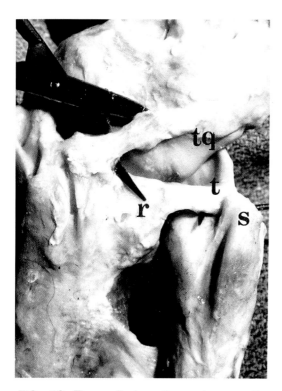

FIG. 12. The radioulnar ligament connection (TFC) and ulnocarpal ligament connection (UTL, ULL) form the so-called triangular fibrocartilage complex (TFCC). Scissors are beneath the dorsal radiotriquetral ligament (distal one-half). The "cup-like" combination of this fibrocartilage and ligament complex extends at the proximal articular surface of the wrist over the ulna, which rotates beneath it. The structure provides both radioulnar and ulnocarpal stability by its strong attachment to the ulnar styloid. r, radius; s, ulnar styloid; tq, triquetrum; t, TFCC.

of the entering scope is the lunotriquetral interosseous ligament (LTL). To the ulnar side and distal is the triquetrum (T), with its surface sloping away distally and volarly. To the radial side distal is the lunate (L) and proximal is the palpably distinct (but visually indistinct) junction between radius and TFC. If the scope is directed ulnarward it can be easily passed into the pisotriquetral recess (b in Fig. 10, Fig. 11) and occasionally into the prestyloid recess. This view is excellent for visualization of the LT ligament, ulnar surface of lunate, triquetral articular surface, TFC, and ulnolunate and ulnotriquetral ligaments. This field of view is shown in Fig. 3 as one would look along arrow 3. Figure 12 shows the major stabilizing ligaments of the distal radioulnar joint and ulnocarpal joint devoid of synovial structures. The important attachments of both the TFC and ulnocarpal ligaments are well seen along with the articular relationships of the ulnar carpal bones.

ARTHROSCOPIC ANATOMY OF THE 6R PORTAL

This portal is located between the extensor digiti minimi (J in Fig. 2) and the extensor carpi ulnaris (ECU) (K in Fig. 2) at the distal margin of the TFC. It is seen photographically marked C in Figs. 7 and 9. Note the relationship of this portal to the portal for the subtriangular fibrocartilage entry into the distal radioulnar joint (portal DRUJ-1). Entry of the scope should be 10° proximal and 10–15° off the vertical toward the center of the radiocarpal joint. You will be entering the ulnocarpal joint over the TFC and its meniscus (if present). The structures seen will be in the relationships noted in Figs. 13 and 14. The lunate's ulnar face and LT ligament will be left and to the top of the visual field in a right wrist,

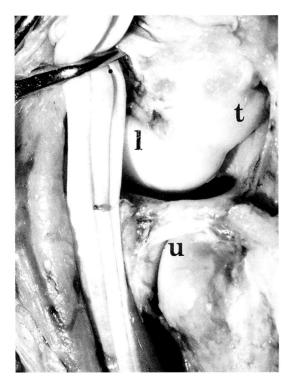

FIG. 13. The ulnocarpal joint is seen grossly from a dorsal ulnar view. The carpal bones are distal [lunate (l), left; triquetrum (t), right], and the ulnar articular dome (u) is seen under the TFC. The ulnotriquetral and ulnolunate ligaments are seen well as one might view them through the 6R portal. Compare with Fig. 14.

with the triquetral articular surface to the top right. The lower surface will be TFC on the left and ulnocarpal ligaments on the right. The TFC will be smooth and soft texturally while the ulnocarpal ligaments will be ligament-like with collagen striations. The meniscal fold

of the ulnocarpal joint will be under the scope, and the latter two will lead the arthroscopic view to the pisotriquetral recess in the extreme upper right of the field. The ulnolunate (UL) and the ulnotriquetral (UT) ligaments are firmly attached to the volar surface of the lunate and triquetrum on their way to further attachments to the capitate and hamate. The two ligaments originate on the ulnar margin of the radius, TFC, and ulnar styloid (in order of increasing importance).

ARTHROSCOPIC ANATOMY OF THE 6U PORTAL

This portal is located on the ulnar margin of the ECU (K in Fig. 2) just distal to the styloid tip (M in Fig. 2). The location of the dorsal sensory branch of the ulnar nerve makes proper entry into this portal important. The use of this portal is usually limited to fluid inflow needles and occasionally a probe. The view through this portal gives one a possible look at the dorsal TFC rim and the adjacent radius (Fig. 15) plus an unparalleled view of the underside of the triquetrum from a directly ulnar view. The lunate and radiocarpal compartments can be seen only with difficulty.

ARTHROSCOPIC ANATOMY OF THE RADIAL MIDCARPAL PORTAL

The radial midcarpal portal lies (Figs. 1–4) approximately 1 cm distal to the 3–4 portal. It is located by palpating the carpal boss (O in Fig. 2) at the base of the axilla between the index and long metacarpals. Move the finger proximally $\frac{1}{2}$ to 1 cm into the depression easily palpable between the distal pole of the scaphoid and the neck of the capitate at the ulnar margin of the ECRB (F in Fig. 2).

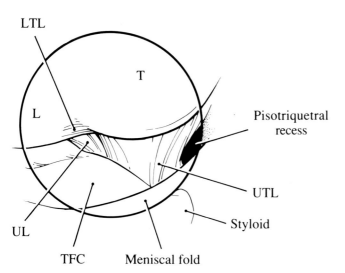

FIG. 14. Arthroscopic view through portal 6R. L, lunate; LTL, lunotriquetral interosseous ligament; T, triquetrum; TFC, triangular fibrocartilage; UL, ulnolunate ligament; UTL, ulnotriquetral ligament.

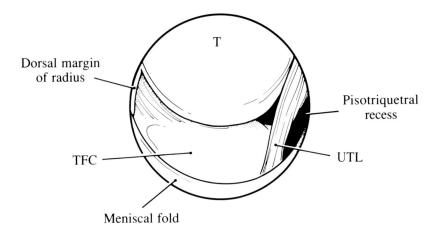

Dorsal margin
of radius

Pisotriquetral
recess

TFC

UTL

Meniscal fold

FIG. 15. Arthroscopic view through portal 6U. The carpus is distal. The ulnotriquetral ligament and pisotriquetral recess are volar (*right*). The view of the meniscal reflexion is variable depending on the depth of the scope and the development of the fold itself. This portal is the only way to view the volar aspect of the triquetral bone and its UCL attachment. T, triquetrum; TFC, triangular fibrocartilage; UTL, ulnotriquetral ligament.

This entry location is well shown in the expanded view of the carpal bones shown in Fig. 3 (arrow 4) and more anatomically in the flexed wrist dissection shown in Fig. 16. The dorsal intercarpal ligaments and dorsal radiotriquetral ligaments are seen well on this specimen. It is possible in a distracted wrist (with good irrigating flow) to pass the scope deep and visualize the continuation of the RSC ligament (depicted in Fig. 3) and to visualize the

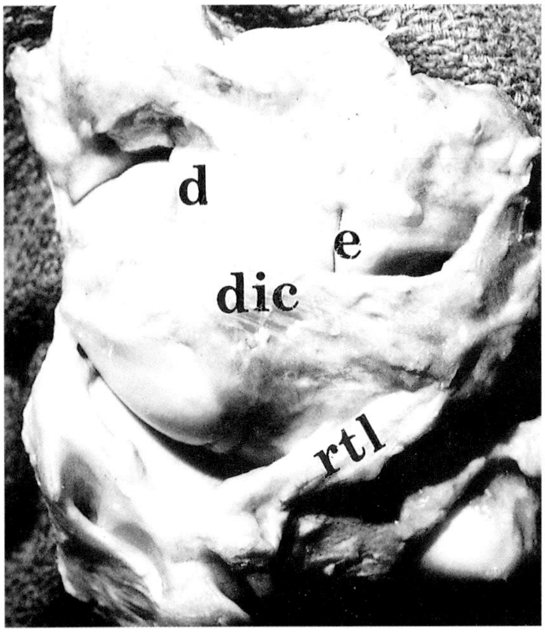

FIG. 16. Gross anatomic view of the midcarpal articulation. The carpus is distal and flexed. The dorsal intercarpal ligament (dic) covers the waist of the scaphoid and distal one-half of the dorsal lunate and joins with the distal radiotriquetral ligament (rtl) over the triquetrum. The radial (d) and ulnar (e) midcarpal portals are shown on either side of the capitate neck at its articulation with the scaphoid radially and the hamate ulnarly.

articular relationships between scaphoid, trapezoid, and trapezium. Passing the scope proximally and ulnarward gives one a midcarpal vantage of the scapholunate articulation with its scapholunate interosseous ligament attached to the two major carpal bones only at their dorsal and volar articular rims, respectively. The opposing articular surfaces of the capitate, scaphoid, and lunate can be seen well. Because of the relatively slack dorsal midcarpal synovial reflection, the scope can be maneuvered over the capitate neck to view the four corners of the capitate, lunate, triquetrum, and hamate, as well as the dorsal one-half of the triquetrohamate articulation (see Figs. 3 and 16).

ARTHROSCOPIC ANATOMY OF THE ULNAR MIDCARPAL PORTAL

For a better view of the lunate triquetral interosseous ligament and volar one-half of the triquetral hamate joint and the triquetral hamate volar ligament use the ulnar midcarpal portal. This portal is located 1 cm distal to the 4–5 portal and about 1.5 cm ulnar to the radial midcarpal portal just at the ulnar margin of the common extensors (I in Fig. 2). The ulnar midcarpal portal lies in line with the central axis of the fourth metacarpal.

The ulnar midcarpal portal is usually used for the introduction of accessory instruments, while viewing through the radial midcarpal portal. However, this portal will accommodate the arthroscope for a clear view of the triquetrohamate joint on the ulnar side, and the articulation of the head of the capitate with the scaphoid and lunate on the radial side.

The ulnar midcarpal portal enters the wrist at the four-corner intersection of the capitate, lunate, triquetrum, and hamate. Looking directly volar from the ulnar midcarpal portal, the continuation of the volar ulnocarpal ligament can be seen representing the ulnar long arm of

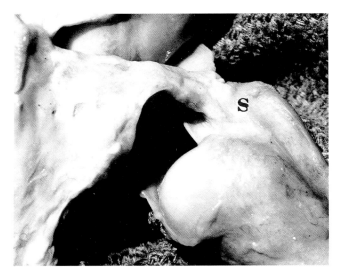

FIG. 17. The distal radioulnar joint opens with the ulna distracted proximally. The TFC remains attached to the ulnar styloid (s). The ligamentum subcruetnum is seen well, as a fold within the joint (see also Fig. 18).

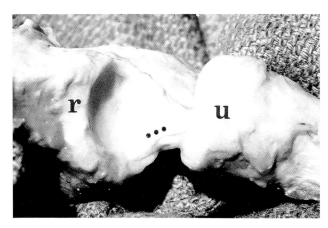

FIG. 18. View of the underside of the TFC. This sigmoid notch is left, the ulna (u) right, and the folded ligamentum subcruetnum (dots) can be seen on the TFC. This fold is flattened against the TFC in pronation and open to lie free within the joint in supination. r, radius.

the volar carpal ligament arch that inserts on the body of the capitate. Inspection of this ligament is especially important in cases of midcarpal instability.

ARTHROSCOPIC ANATOMY OF THE STT PORTAL

The third useful portal for the midcarpal space lies directly over the dorsal aspect of the scaphotrapeziotrapezoid (STT) articulation. The STT portal is located in line with the midshaft axis of the second metacarpal, just ulnar to the extensor policis longus tendon. Entry into this portal requires traction on the index finger. The STT portal is used primarily as an accessory portal to address articular lesions on the distal pole of the scaphoid, or to decompress the STT joint in advanced arthritic conditions. Leaving the extensor policis longus tendon to the radial side of the STT portal protects the radial artery from injury as it courses toward the base of the first metacarpal.

ARTHROSCOPIC ANATOMY OF THE DISTAL RADIOULNAR JOINT PORTALS

Portal DRUJ-1 is located immediately proximal to the 6R portal (Fig. 2, arrow 5 in Fig. 3, small sharp probe in Fig. 12, and d in Fig. 9). A gross view of this entry area is

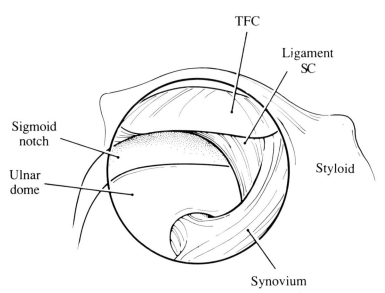

FIG. 19. Arthroscopic view from portal DRUJ-1. The structures seen are with a shallow penetration of the arthroscope. The radial face of the ulnar articular surface cannot be seen. This angle gives a good view of the ulnar dome articular chondromalacia seen in the impingement syndromes. Compare this view with the anatomic representations in Figs. 17 and 18. TFC, triangular fibrocartilage; SC, ligament subcruetnum.

shown in Figs. 17 and 18. As the scope enters the articular cavity the ligamentum subcruetnum may be encountered, depending on the position of rotation of the wrist (prominent in supination and folded flat in pronation). The scope will view the dome of the articular surface of the ulna. This surface faces the underside of the TFC. The distant face of cartilage is the sigmoid notch (Fig. 19). Portal distal radioulnar joint 2 (DRUJ-2) is in the axilla of the radius and ulna and entry here will provide a view of the proximal sigmoid notch cartilage and its adjacent ulnar articular cartilage.

REFERENCES

1. Bowers WH. The distal radioulnar joint. In: Green DP, ed. *Operative hand surgery.* 2nd Ed. Vol. 1. New York: Churchill Livingstone, 1988, pp. 939–990.
2. Green DP. Carpal dislocations and instabilities. In: Green DP, ed. *Operative hand surgery.* 2nd Ed. Vol. 1. New York: Churchill Livingstone, 1988, pp. 815–938.
3. Lichtman DM. *The wrist and its disorders.* Philadelphia: WB Saunders, 1988.
4. Palmer AK. Fracture of the distal radius. In: Green DP, ed. *Operative hand surgery.* 2nd Ed. Vol. 1. New York: Churchill Livingstone, 1988, pp. 991–1026.
5. Taleisnik, J. *The wrist.* New York: Churchill Livingstone, 1985.

CHAPTER 3

Imaging of the Wrist

Thomas L. Pope, Jr., M.D., *Gary G. Poehling*, M.D., *David B. Siegel*, M.D., *and Michael Y. M. Chen*, M.D.

Interestingly, the hand and wrist were the first body parts to be radiographed when in 1895 Wilhelm Conrad Roentgen, a professor of physics at the University of Wurzburg, Germany, produced a radiographic image of his wife's hand. The wrist is a complex anatomic region and wrist pain may result from a variety of factors. The initial diagnostic evaluation of wrist symptoms, as with any clinical problem, comprises a thorough history and complete physical examination. An integral part of this evaluation is to relate the point of maximal tenderness in an individual carpal bone or ligamentous region so that the appropriate imaging tests can be selected. The arthroscopist should be familiar with the normal anatomy of the wrist and the wide range of imaging choices available for its evaluation, should know some of the limitations and strengths of each examination, and should have a logical plan for requesting examinations in vari-

ous clinical situations. This approach will minimize patient discomfort and maximize both the diagnostic yield and the cost–benefit of the examinations.

This chapter discusses the imaging "shopping list" of diagnostic modalities available to the orthopaedist and arthroscopist, stresses the importance of technique in the evaluation of wrist abnormalities, summarizes the basic normal radiographic anatomy of the wrist, and suggests a rational algorithmic approach that should maximize diagnostic yield in some of the common wrist disorders requiring arthroscopy.

IMAGING "SHOPPING LIST"

Table 1 lists the wide range of imaging tests available to the arthroscopist to evaluate the wrist. Because there

17

TABLE 1. *Imaging "shopping list"*

Plain films
Tomography
Fluoroscopy
Computed tomography (CT)
Arthrography
   Single contrast
   Double contrast
   CT arthrography
Magnetic resonance (MR) imaging
Ultrasound
Nuclear medicine

is a substantial difference in the cost of these examinations, it is imperative that the potential yield be considered before the test is requested or performed. For example, ultrasound would be inappropriate for evaluating a suspected tear in the triangular fibrocartilage complex (TFCC) because it cannot image this structure well, but arthrography (single- or triple-joint injection) or magnetic resonance (MR) imaging would be an appropriate test to use because either can show the integrity of this anatomic region.

The relative strengths and weaknesses of each of the examinations in Table 1 depend on the patient's clinical situation; some of these strengths and weaknesses are outlined in the individual sections. The precise clinical role of many of these imaging tests in the evaluation of wrist abnormalities is currently under review in clinical trials. In every situation, however, after the history is obtained and the physical examination performed, the plain radiograph is the first appropriate imaging examination in the workup of wrist problems.

TECHNIQUE AND ANATOMY OF THE ROUTINE PLAIN-FILM EXAMINATION

Information gained from the plain-film evaluation of the wrist often determines whether, and if so, which, further diagnostic studies are necessary. Excellent technique is imperative because suboptimal films are a common cause of misinterpretation (7,26).

The routine radiographic examination of the wrist varies among institutions and radiologists. At a minimum, the posteroanterior (PA) and lateral projections with the x-ray beam centered on the wrist are required for adequate assessment of the uncomplicated wrist problem. In some instances, a radiopaque marker designating the point of maximal pain and tenderness may be helpful in determining the site of radiographic abnormality.

Posteroanterior View

The PA view should be obtained with the forearm in neutral rotation by abducting the arm 90° from the chest and flexing the elbow approximately 90°. The patient should sit on a chair or stool beside the table in a position that allows comfortable placement of the hand and wrist palm down on the x-ray cassette or table surface. This method will ensure a true PA projection (Fig. 1A and B).

On the PA view, the soft tissues should be evaluated

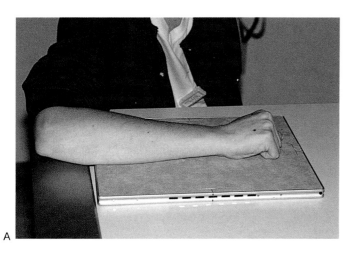
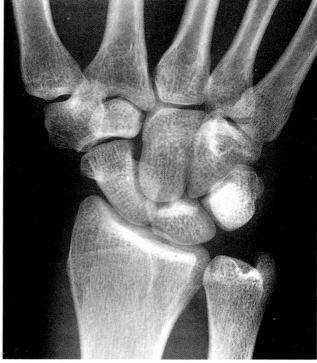

FIG. 1. A: PA view of wrist. Standard positioning for the PA view of the wrist. Note the slightly clenched fist. **B:** Normal PA radiograph of the wrist.

first (31,51). The scaphoid fat plane or stripe, a thin radiolucent line paralleling the lateral scaphoid surface, is the most important soft-tissue landmark on the PA view (Fig. 2). Hemorrhage or edema may cause obliteration of this line (Fig. 3) and may be the only sign of acute scaphoid fracture (24,32,138). Three smoothly curving parallel lines, called ARCs, define the normal relationship of the distal radioulnar joint to the proximal carpal row and the proximal carpal row to the midcarpal row (51) (Fig. 4). ARC I follows the convex surfaces of the scaphoid, lunate, and triquetrum, and ARC II outlines the distal curve of these same three bones. ARC III, the most distal curve, is defined by the proximal curvatures of the capitate and hamate bones. Discontinuity of these arcs or overlapping carpal bones usually represents carpal malalignment (51).

All the joint spaces demonstrated on the normal PA view should be approximately equal in width and should measure 1–2 mm. Widening of any of these spaces to 4 mm or more—most commonly encountered at the scapholunate joint—usually indicates ligamentous disruption (Fig. 5), although increased joint fluid and synovial hypertrophy are other possible causes. Narrowing of these spaces follows arthritic change, traumatic joint disruption, or carpal coalition (Fig. 6).

The scaphoid, lunate, and triquetrum bones have typical configurations on the PA view in palmar flexion and dorsiflexion. If one bone is out of phase with the other

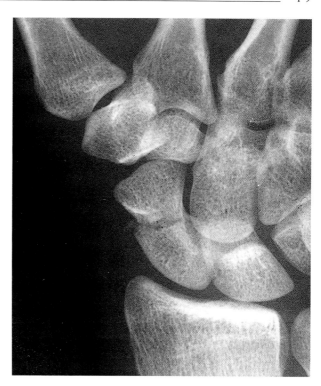

FIG. 3. Loss of navicular fat stripe. PA view of right wrist of a patient with navicular fracture shows obliteration of the navicular fat stripe.

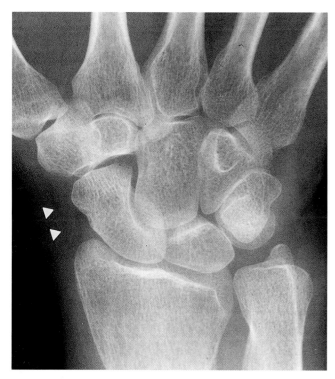

FIG. 2. Navicular fat stripe. Normal PA view of wrist with soft-tissue technique highlighting the navicular fat stripe (*white arrowheads*).

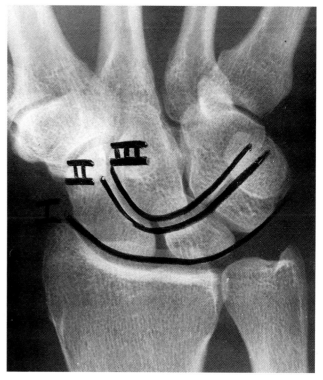

FIG. 4. Normal wrist relationship. PA view of right wrist shows the three symmetric carpal arcs first described by Gilula (51).

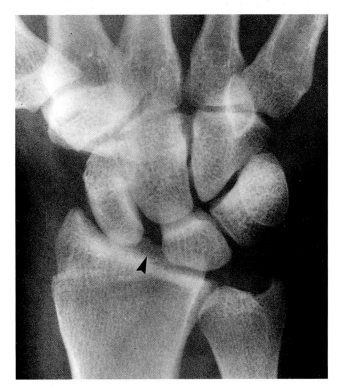

FIG. 5. Scapholunate dissociation. Normal PA view of right wrist shows widening of the scapholunate junction (*arrowhead*).

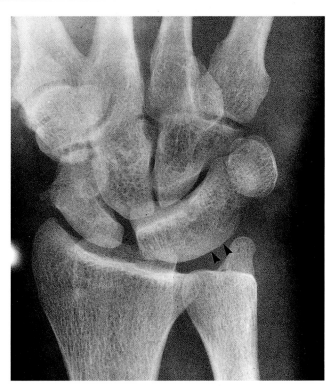

FIG. 6. Congenital fusion. PA view of right wrist showing congenital fusion of the lunate and triquetrum (*arrowheads*).

two, an intrinsic interosseous ligamentous disruption should be suspected. A few technical points regarding positioning and the appearance of the scaphoid on the PA view should be stressed. In the normal PA view, the scaphoid bone is roughly triangular, and its joint surfaces parallel those of the trapezium, the capitate, and the lunate bones. With radial deviation or palmar flexion, the normal scaphoid is flexed palmarly and becomes foreshortened on the PA film, producing a "signet ring" appearance. This may be misinterpreted as rotatory scaphoid subluxation. However, in foreshortening caused by positioning alone, the scapholunate space should be normal (Fig. 7). The lunate bone becomes triangular with palmar flexion and the triquetrum slides down the hamate. With ulnar deviation, the scaphoid bone normally becomes elongated on the PA view by dorsiflexing the wrist, while the lunate becomes quadrangular and the triquetrum engages the hamate distally (Fig. 8).

The PA view also shows the relationship of the distal radius and ulna. The ulnar styloid process is positioned directly opposite the radius, and the distal articulating surfaces of both the ulna and radius form a smooth concentric arc (Fig. 9). Variation of this normal relationship is termed "ulnar variance" and may predispose to certain predictable pathologic conditions (see pathologic conditions of the distal radioulnar joint later in this chapter) (146).

Lateral View

The lateral wrist view is obtained with the humerus adducted against the chest wall and the forearm in neutral rotation. The ulnar side of the hand and wrist should be placed flush against the radiographic cassette to ensure that the forearm and dorsum of the hand are in alignment without rotation. In the properly positioned lateral view, the distal ulna should project directly over the midportion of the radius and the pisiform should be visualized (Fig. 10).

The most important soft tissue landmark on the lateral view is the pronator quadratus fat pad (Fig. 10B). Displacement of this structure may indicate an underlying pathologic condition (32,138); also, soft tissue swelling on the dorsum of the hand and wrist is best appreciated in this view. The bony relationships on the lateral view are best evaluated by the following relationships: a nearly straight line should be formed by connecting the midportion of the third metacarpal (which is tightly fixed to the distal aspect of the capitate), the rounded head of the capitate (which fits snugly within the distal lunate concavity), and the proximal lunate (which is nestled within the concavity of the distal radius) (Fig. 11). The normal angulation of this line averages 10° in most cases (5,51). The scapholunate, capitolunate, and radioscaphoid angles also should be reviewed. The normal scapholunate

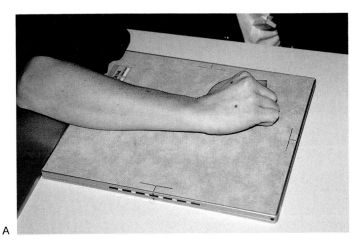

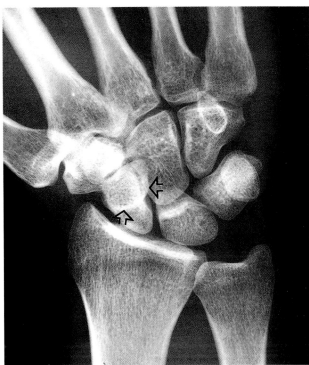

FIG. 7. A: Standard technique for obtaining radial deviation of wrist. **B:** PA radiograph of the right wrist taken in radial deviation showing the signet ring appearance of the scaphoid (*arrows*) in this position. This should not be misinterpreted as rotatory subluxation.

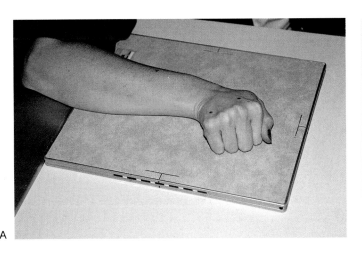

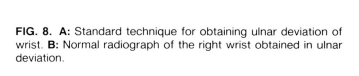

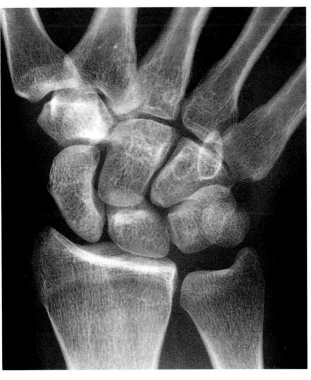

FIG. 8. A: Standard technique for obtaining ulnar deviation of wrist. **B:** Normal radiograph of the right wrist obtained in ulnar deviation.

angle ranges from 30° to 60° (Fig. 12), the capitolunate angle from 0° to 30° (Fig. 13), and the radioscaphoid angle from 121° to 150° (Fig. 14). Of these, the most important one to check is the scapholunate angle (30,51,54,66).

The lateral view also shows the normal relationship of the distal radioulnar joint, in which the radius and ulna directly overlap on this view (Fig. 10). Minimal degrees of supination and pronation can make evaluation of this articulation difficult, and computed tomography (CT) is recommended for definitive diagnosis (see Pathology section).

Oblique Views

Oblique views usually are reserved for evaluating acute trauma or confirming an abnormality suggested on the standard PA and lateral projections. Views are obtained with 45° of rotation from the standard PA view (Fig. 15). The main advantage of the oblique views is to decrease the overlap of the individual carpal bones that is present on the PA and lateral films.

SUPPLEMENTAL PLAIN-FILM EXAMINATIONS

Due to the bony overlap normally present in the routine wrist series, a number of supplemental plain-film

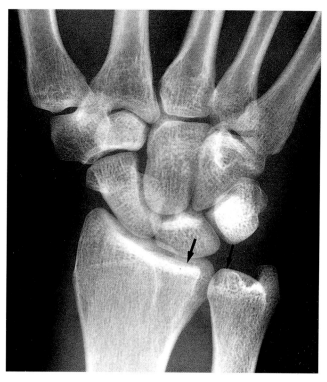

FIG. 9. Normal radius/ulnar relationship. PA view of wrist showing the normal relationship of distal radius and ulna (*arrows*). The distal radius and the distal ulna should be approximately equal in length in the normal situation.

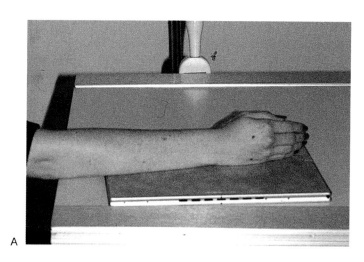

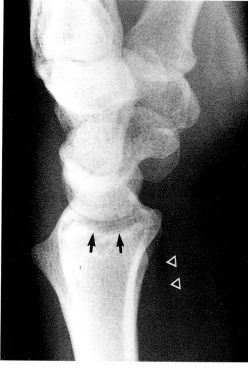

FIG. 10. A: Standard technique for obtaining lateral view of the wrist. B: Lateral radiograph of the wrist showing the pronator quadratus fat stripe (*white arrowheads*) and the concavity of the distal radius (*arrows*).

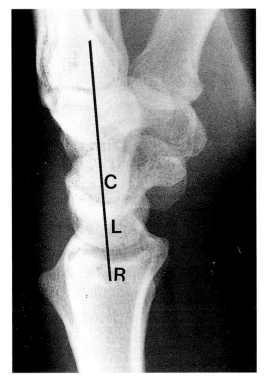

FIG. 11. Normal lateral wrist relationship. Lateral radiograph of wrist showing linear relationship of distal radius (R), lunate (L), and capitate (C).

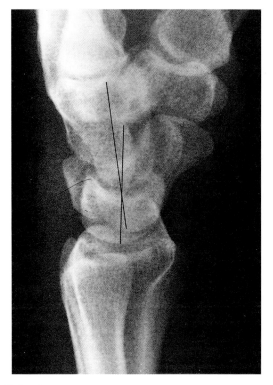

FIG. 13. Normal capitolunate angle. Lateral view of wrist showing normal capitolunate angle.

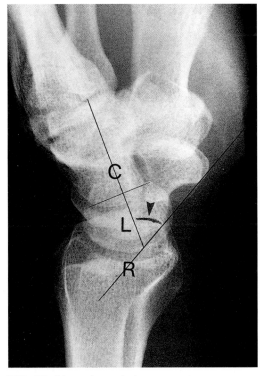

FIG. 12. Normal scapholunate angle. Lateral radiograph of wrist showing normal scapholunate angle of 45° (*arrowhead*). C, capitate; L, lunate; R, radius.

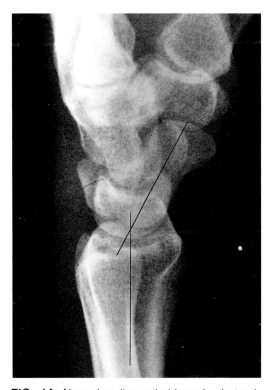

FIG. 14. Normal radioscaphoid angle. Lateral view of wrist showing normal radioscaphoid angle.

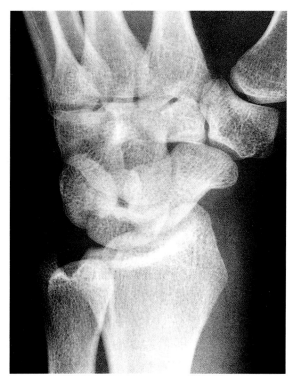

FIG. 15. Oblique view of wrist. Normal oblique radiograph of the wrist.

views have been recommended for better evaluation of individual carpal bones or the relationships between them. The appropriateness of these examinations should be determined from the findings of the history and physical examination or from suspicious areas on the routine plain-film examination.

Scaphoid

Scaphoid views are indicated when pain in the region of the anatomic "snuff box" is suggestive of scaphoid bone lesions. These views are obtained by ulnarly deviating the hand or by angling the x-ray tube 45° cranially (Fig. 16). These maneuvers elongate and profile the long axis of the scaphoid (Fig. 17). Alternatively, Stecher suggested that the "clenched-fist view," which pronates the hand and produces carpal loading, may increase the diagnostic yield by widening the scaphoid fracture line (132) (Fig. 18). Other authors have proposed ulnar deviation to improve fracture visualization, although this maneuver may have the potentially harmful effect of distracting the fracture fragments (56,122).

Hamate

Specialized views are necessary for adequate visualization of the hook of the hamate. The carpal tunnel view,

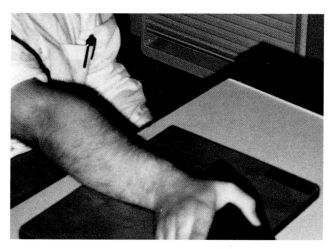

FIG. 16. Scaphoid view. Standard positioning for scaphoid view of the wrist. Note the use of the wedge and the abduction of the thumb.

first described by Hart and Gaynor (61), gives an axial end-on view of the carpal canal. This study is performed with the pronated forearm on the x-ray cassette and the patient manually dorsiflexing the hand by pulling the fingertips dorsally with the other hand. The x-ray beam angle is 25° to 35° and is directed to the volar carpal surface. Alternatively, the palm of the hand may be placed on the cassette and the wrist hyperextended. The degree

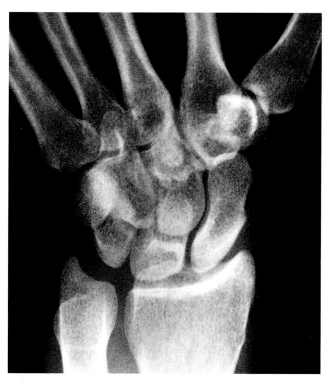

FIG. 17. Normal radiograph of the scaphoid showing its elongated appearance on this view.

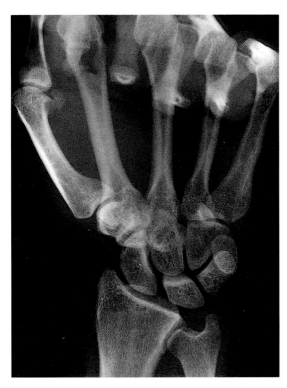

FIG. 18. Stecher's clenched-fist view of the wrist.

of central beam angulation then depends on the degree of hyperextension. This projection is especially effective in diagnosing fractures of the hook of the hamate and the trapezial ridge and in evaluating the integrity of the pisiform–triquetrum joint (1,155) (Fig. 19).

Trapezium

An adequate view of the trapezium also often requires special projections. Boyes described a palm-down 35° view with the wrist in ulnar deviation and the thumb adducted and extended to best display this bone (16). However, Bowers suggests that a more effective method is to place the wrist in the lateral projection with the elbow raised from the cassette (15). The beam is centered at the scaphotrapezium–trapezoid joint with the thumb extended and abducted and the hand slightly pronated. Bowers called this projection the "Bette view" (Fig. 20).

Pisiform

The pisiform, a sesamoid bone within the flexor carpi ulnaris tendon, can be seen on the carpal tunnel view. Moneim described a semisupinated off-lateral projection that profiles the pisiform, hook of the hamate, and piso-triquetral joint (95) (Fig. 21).

FLUOROSCOPY

All the routine and supplemental wrist examinations described above are obtained with standard radiographic equipment. In some patients, however, there may still be unanswered questions. In such cases, fluoroscopic examination of the wrist may be helpful in the detection of subtle nondisplaced fractures, subtle abnormalities of the trapezio–first metacarpal joint, and ligamentous abnormalities. Abnormal kinematics are usually manifested by a "snap" in the wrist with sudden shift of the carpal bones under fluoroscopy. Fluoroscopy is particularly helpful in the evaluation of carpal instability (17,52,53,76,111,123,135,153).

TOMOGRAPHY

The major applications of tomography in the upper extremity are to delineate the true extent of known distal radial or carpal fractures, to detect subtle nondisplaced carpal fractures (especially of the scaphoid and hamate), and to delineate the degree of malunion, particularly in scaphoid fractures (3,29,126). With standard tomographic technique, sections are obtained at intervals of 2–3 mm and angles of 90°. In the wrist, 1-mm intervals may be required for subtle abnormalities. The positioning of the patient for tomography depends on the finding on plain films and ideally tomography should be supervised, monitored, and tailored by the person who will interpret the tomograms (Fig. 22).

ULTRASOUND

The primary use of ultrasound is the evaluation of soft-tissue abnormalities. For example, ultrasound can be helpful in the evaluation of palpable soft-tissue lesions to determine whether they are cystic or solid, in the setting of possible soft-tissue infection to delineate abscess cavities, in the evaluation of the carpal tunnel, and, occasionally, in confirming a clinical diagnosis of tenosynovitis (46,68,128). The future for ultrasound may include evaluation of partial tendon lacerations or erosions and vascular abnormalities, although these indications are still in the investigational stage.

RADIONUCLIDE IMAGING

Radionuclide bone imaging (nuclear scintigraphy) is also referred to as the nuclear medicine "bone scan" and is an extremely sensitive technique. This sensitivity makes radionuclide imaging an excellent means of establishing the location of the abnormality in patients with pain who have normal plain films (134). This feature is particularly important in the diagnosis of subtle scaph-

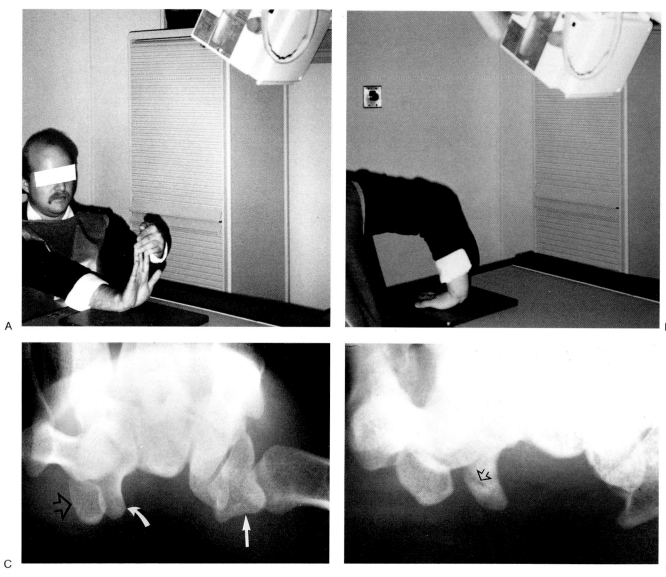

FIG. 19. **A and B:** Alternative techniques for obtaining a carpal tunnel view of the wrist. Either of these techniques may be used for this projection. **C:** Carpal tunnel view radiograph showing the pisiform (*open arrow*), the hamate (*curved arrow*), and the trapezium (*straight arrow*). **D:** Carpal tunnel view showing minimally displaced fracture of the hook of the hamate (*open arrow*).

oid and hamate fractures and stress fractures which, in the wrist, most commonly occur in the ulnae of young athletes (Fig. 23) (82–84,97,118–121,131).

Finally, the use of bone scanning has also been described in the evaluation of infection, primary bone lesions (especially osteoid osteoma), avascular necrosis (especially of the lunate; Kienböch's disease), reflex sympathetic dystrophy (RSD) (Fig. 24), and fracture healing (40,79,88,127,148).

ARTHROGRAPHY

Arthrography (radiography after intraarticular injection of contrast medium) is used for direct evaluation of

the status of the intrasynovial intercarpal ligaments and TFCC or for indirect examination of the integrity of the intracapsular extrasynovial ligaments (47,92). The major indications for arthrography are listed in Table 2. Early reports of wrist arthrography described injection solely into the radiocarpal joint (RCJ) under fluoroscopic guidance; films were obtained immediately after confirmation that the injection was intraarticular (73). The importance of continuous fluoroscopic control during the injection of contrast material and exercise was later stressed in the literature (53). After injection into the RCJ, there is normally no communication between this space and the midcarpal joint (MCJ) or the distal radioulnar joint (DRUJ), although the incidence of communication increases with age (117). In 1985, Tirman

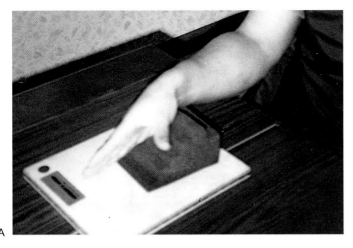

A

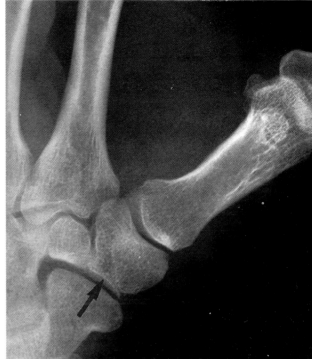

B

FIG. 20. A: Bette view. Standard technique for obtaining the Bette view of the trapezium. **B:** Normal Bette view showing excellent visualization of the trapezium (*arrow*).

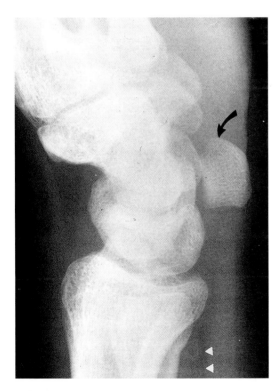

FIG. 21. Semisupinated view of wrist. Radiograph of wrist taken in semisupinated position shows the pisiform projected away from the remainder of the carpal bones (*curved arrow*). The pronator quadratus fat pad may also be seen in this view (*white arrowheads*).

suggested that any RCJ and MCJ communications might best be evaluated by injection of the contrast agent into the MCJ (140). Subsequently, a triple-compartment technique requiring injection into the RCJ, MCJ, and DRUJ was reported (74). This study can be performed in a single sitting with the use of digital subtraction technique or by using different concentrations of contrast medium (28,80,100,110,117). The majority of institutions, however, perform the study by first injecting the RCJ and then having the patient return 2 to 3 hours later to have the MCJ and DRUJ injections.

The advantage of the triple-injection technique is reported to be the demonstration of one-way, or "ball valve," communications between the wrist compartments in up to one-fourth of patients (74,75). However, the experience at other institutions shows that one-way communications occur in less than 10% of patients, and no distinct advantage is gained with the triple-joint injection technique (81,154). At the present time, the most rational approach appears to be close communication between the radiologist and orthopaedist in deciding which of these examinations is most appropriate in a given clinical situation. Further research into the efficacy of the two techniques is needed to determine the advantages of one method over the other.

At our institution, both single RCJ injection and triple-compartment injection with digital fluoroscopy and subtraction are used, and the choice depends on the clinical situation. Both ionic and nonionic contrast media are used, according to the preference of the radiolo-

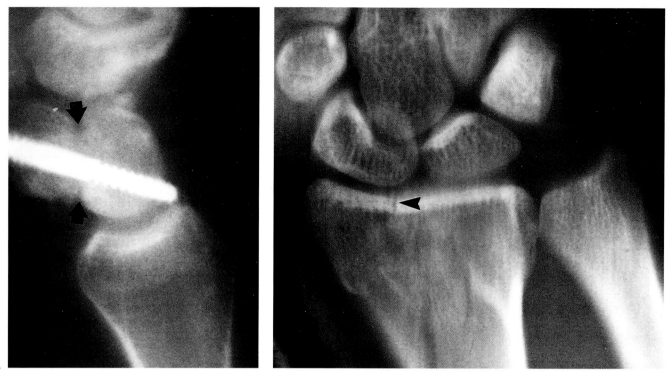

FIG. 22. The value of tomography. **A:** Lateral tomogram of a navicular fracture treated with Herbert's screw shows nonhealing of the navicular waist fracture (*arrows*). **B:** PA tomogram of different patient with comminuted fracture of the distal radius on plain films shows unsuspected intraarticular involvement (*arrowhead*).

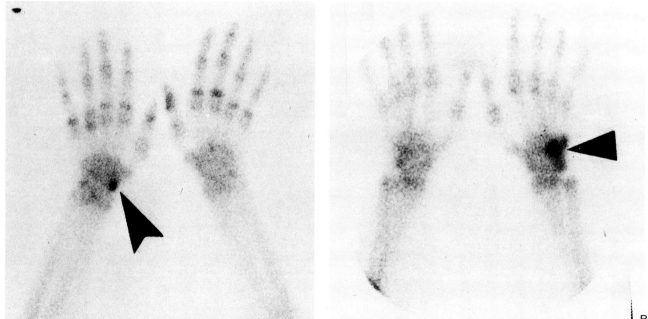

FIG. 23. Radionuclide bone scan. **A:** PA view of wrist and hands shows focal area of increased uptake in the region of the scaphoid, representing a scaphoid fracture not appreciated on the plain films. **B:** PA view of hands and wrist from radionuclide bone scan in a different patient shows increased radionuclide tracer localization in the lateral aspect of the right hand representing an unsuspected hamate fracture.

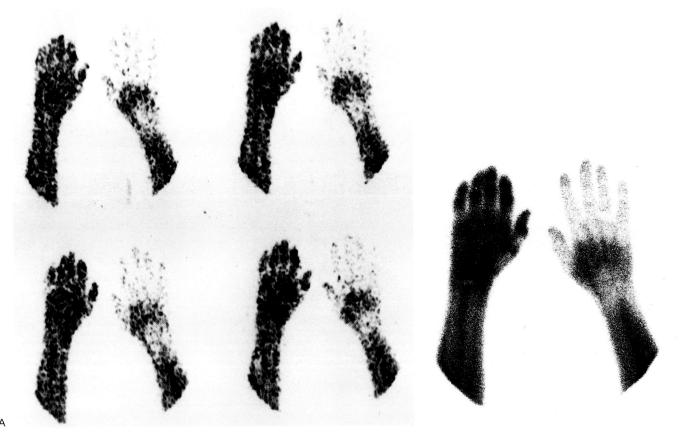

A

B

FIG. 24. Reflex sympathetic dystrophy (RSD). **A:** PA palms down view of radionuclide bone scan in patient with symptoms of RSD shows diffuse increased radionuclide tracer localization in the right hand. **B:** This increased localization persists on the delayed views and is compatible with RSD. (Courtesy of Dr. Nat Watson, The Bowman Gray School of Medicine, Wake Forest University.)

gist. Nonionic media have the advantages of less risk of anaphylaxis and less patient discomfort during and after the examination. However, either medium is acceptable because of the extremely low incidence of reactions to intraarticular contrast injections.

In the normal wrist arthrogram, there is no intercarpal communication between the RCJ, MCJ, and DRUJ compartments. A prominent prestyloid recess located on

the ulnar aspect of the RCJ compartment at the tip of the ulnar styloid process and excrescences on the volar side of the joint are commonly encountered and represent normal variation (Fig. 25).

Isolated communications between the radiocarpal and midcarpal compartments increase with age and have been reported in 13% to 47% of cases. These communications usually are bilateral and symmetric, and must be correlated with the patient's age and physical activity (35). With a cadaver study, Mikic showed that perforation never occurred in the fetus or during the first and second decades and that degeneration and perforation of the compartments were more common with aging (91). In a clinical study, Trentham reviewed 200 wrist arthrograms in a random population aged 40 to 90 years and found that RCJ and MCJ communications increased with age in up to 47% of patients (142). In a prospective trial of bilateral arthrography in patients with wrist pain, Herbert et al. found that 74% of the patients had positive arthrograms even in the asymptomatic wrist (62). Therefore, the finding of a ligamentous perforation on arthrography, especially a communication between the RCJ and

---

TABLE 2. *Indications for arthrography of the wrist*

1. Persistent wrist pain with "normal" plain films
2. Suspected disruption of triangular fibrocartilage
   A. With fracture
   B. Without fracture
3. Differentiating fibrous union from nonunion of the navicular
4. Ganglia
5. Congenital deformities
6. Inflammatory arthropathies
7. Miscellaneous—loose bodies, suspected pigmented villonodular synovitis, giant synovial cysts, and so forth

From Dalinka, ref. 34, with permission.

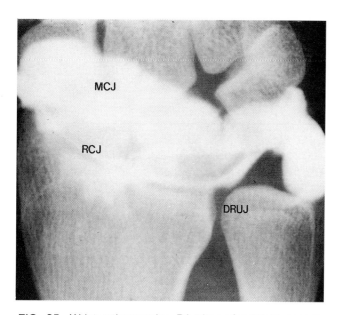

FIG. 25. Wrist arthrography. PA view of wrist in normal single-contrast arthrogram with injection into the radiocarpal joint (RCJ) showing no communication with the distal radioulnar joint (DRUJ) or with the midcarpal joint (MCJ).

MCJ compartments, must be correlated with the patient's symptoms because it may be secondary to degeneration and have no functional significance.

In decreasing order, the most common sites of clinically significant compartmental communications seen on wrist arthrography are by way of the scapholunate ligament, the lunotriquetral ligament, and the TFCC (103). Other sites of communication do occur, but rarely are thought to be of clinical importance (Fig. 26).

COMPUTED TOMOGRAPHY

Computed tomography (CT) can play an important role in evaluating wrist disorders. Thin slices (1.5–2.0 mm) in both the transaxial and the coronal planes are necessary for best results (112). Transaxial imaging with thin slices followed by reconstruction in the sagittal or coronal planes is the preferred procedure at some institutions. Direct coronal and sagittal acquisitions also can be obtained with appropriate positioning.

The major indications and applications of CT are in suspected dislocations of the radioulnar joint, fracture follow-up and evaluation of healing, subtle or complex fracture evaluation (particularly of the hamate), diagnosis of intraarticular loose bodies, and soft-tissue injury

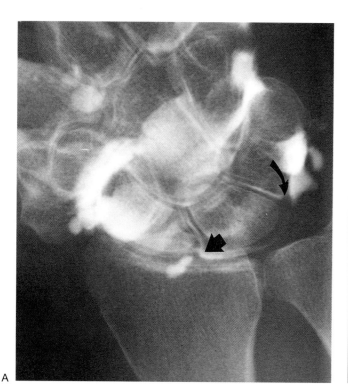

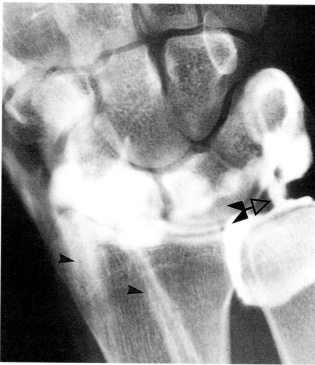

A

B

FIG. 26. A: Scapholunate ligament tear. PA radial deviation view of arthrogram after RCJ injection shows a tear of the scapholunate ligament diagnosed by communication of the RCJ with the MCJ (*arrow*). Note the intact lunotriquetral ligament (*curved arrow*). **B:** TFCC tear by arthrography. PA view of wrist arthrogram after RCJ injection shows communication of the RCJ with the DRUJ through a tear of the TFCC (*arrow*). Note iatrogenic injection of contrast into tendon sheaths (*arrowheads*).

or disease (22,41,63,72,93,94,99,101,106,112,114,124, 137,149,160). CT arthrography has recently been advocated to supplement conventional arthrography, and early experience with 3D CT in surgical planning and evaluation of subtle abnormalities has been promising (9,10,18,42,98,113). Stress CT also has been advocated for determining translational motion of the radioulnar joint (109).

MAGNETIC RESONANCE IMAGING

Magnetic resonance (MR) imaging is an exciting technique with a broad range of potential uses in wrist examinations because it is noninvasive, uses no radiation, and provides excellent soft-tissue contrast and detail. As with all musculoskeletal MR imaging, surface coils and small field-of-view imaging are mandatory for the best diagnostic results. MR imaging is the only noninvasive technique that can depict intricate soft-tissue anatomy and hyaline cartilage; therefore, it holds much promise in the preoperative evaluation of wrist disorders (6,12,71,90,115,141,150).

The major indications for MR imaging of the wrist are in the evaluation of avascular necrosis of the lunate and scaphoid bones, TFCC tears, carpal ligamentous disruption, soft-tissue lesions in the vicinity of the wrist, and carpal tunnel syndrome (4,11,25,37,55,59,86,89,116, 125,129,133,143,158,159).

In summary, a wide range of diagnostic techniques is at the disposal of the arthroscopist. For the majority of patients, however, an in-depth history, thorough physical examination, and plain radiographs will direct the imaging workup. Although many questions can be answered by special plain-film views coupled with fluoroscopy, a number of patients will require further evaluation.

Proper utilization of these supplemental tests, some of which are extremely expensive, requires a basic understanding of the technique of the examination and its strengths and weaknesses, as well as close cooperation and communication between the orthopaedist and the radiologist. A basic algorithm for selecting certain tests is shown in Fig. 27.

For suspected ligamentous disruption, arthrography is probably the best preoperative test, although it does have a 30% to 40% false-positive rate. In findings compatible with TFCC tears, either arthrography or MR imaging is acceptable, and further investigation may show a slight advantage for MR due to the additional information it provides. For subtle fractures, CT is still the best technique, but if avascular necrosis is the clinical concern, MR imaging is the most appropriate investigational tool. For suspected soft-tissue abnormalities such as tumors,

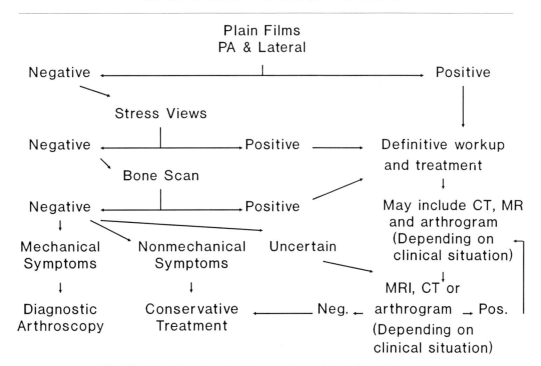

FIG. 27. Algorithm for selecting supplemental studies of the wrist.

infection, or nerve entrapment, MR imaging is the preferred imaging modality at the present time. However, these recommendations may vary according to the availability and cost of the procedure, as well as the experience and interpretive skills of the radiologist. Therefore, it is the responsibility of the surgeon to be aware of the strengths and weaknesses of each modality at any particular institution.

NORMAL VARIATION

Congenital and normal variations are commonly encountered in the wrist. Separate ossification centers such as the os styloideum are not uncommon and are best demonstrated in the semisupinated or internal oblique projections (Fig. 28). These structures are important because they may be interpreted as pathologic lesions. Congenital fusions also may be seen and usually do not cause diagnostic difficulties (Fig. 6).

In cases of suspected normal variation, Keats' *Atlas of Normal Roentgen Variants That May Simulate Disease* or Kohler's *Borderlands of the Normal and Early Pathologic Findings in Skeletal Radiography* should be consulted.

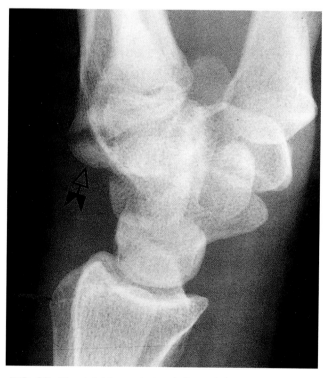

FIG. 28. Os styloideum. Lateral view of the wrist in patient with palpable lump between second and third metacarpals, which was thought clinically to be a fracture at the base of the metacarpals. The os styloideum, an ossicle lying between the capitate and the base of the second and third metacarpals, produces the small immovable protuberance noted on the dorsum of the hand, which may be confused as a fracture.

WRIST ABNORMALITIES

Carpal Bone Fractures

Trauma to the distal forearm, usually resulting from a fall on an outstretched arm and hand, may cause a variety of fractures and dislocations of the distal radius and individual carpal bones, or a combination of fractures, dislocations, and ligamentous injury (38). The majority of these bony injuries are diagnosed at the initial presentation by routine plain-film radiography. In certain situations, however, CT may be needed to clarify the extent and relationship of bony injuries in an acute fracture. The advantages of CT are (a) planar imaging, which eliminates the difficulties that overlapping structures present within the wrist, and (b) the choice of axial, oblique, sagittal, or coronal imaging planes to best define the bony anatomy (Fig. 29).

In patients with chronic pain and normal plain films, the radionuclide bone scan is an excellent screening test for subtle fractures. Once an area of abnormal uptake is identified on the bone scan, specialized plain-film views and CT are recommended for further evaluation. The most common carpal fractures are those of the scaphoid, triquetrum, lunate, and hamate structures, although isolated fractures of the other carpal bones occur on rare occasions (87) (Figs. 23 and 24).

Scaphoid Fractures

The scaphoid bone is located in a unique position, bridging the proximal and distal carpal rows and adding mobility and stability to the wrist. However, this bone is prone to fracture, and in persons between the ages of 15 and 40 years it accounts for about 80% of fractures of the carpal bones. Typically, these fractures result from a fall on the outstretched hand (39). Tenderness in the anatomic snuff box is the characteristic physical finding associated with this injury. The majority of scaphoid fractures (about 70%) occur through the anatomic waist because of the extreme stress placed on this area during forced dorsiflexion (144) (see Figs. 3 and 30). Twenty percent of scaphoid fractures occur in the proximal pole and the remainder in the distal pole (87) (Fig. 31). Associated injuries are fractures of the capitate, radial styloid process, and triquetrum, as well as perilunate dislocation. Scaphoid fractures may be subtle and may not be identified on the initial plain-film examination, even with scaphoid views. In patients with persistent pain, a radionuclide bone scan may be a worthwhile screening study, and CT also is a good alternative (107) (see Fig. 27).

Proximal waist or proximal pole fractures predispose the scaphoid to delayed union or nonunion, as well as

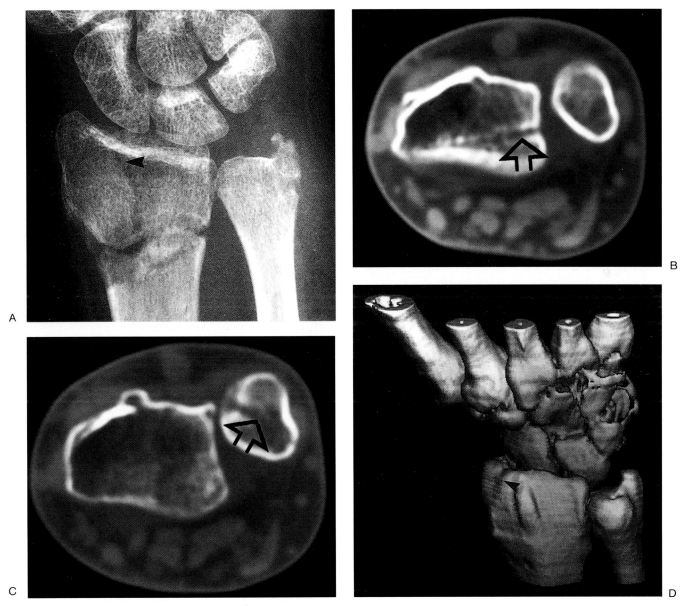

FIG. 29. Distal radial fracture. **A:** Plain film of distal radial and ulnar styloid fractures showing suspected intraarticular extent (*arrowhead*). **B:** Axial CT image confirms fracture extending through to the ulnar side of the radius (*open arrow*). **C:** Slightly more distal axial CT image shows the oblique fracture through the distal ulna to better advantage (*open arrow*). **D:** 3D CT image of the same patient in the oblique position shows the intraarticular fracture of the distal radius (*arrowhead*). The advantage of 3D CT imaging is that the exact relationship of the fracture fragments can be appreciated, and this technique holds promise in the future for better surgical planning.

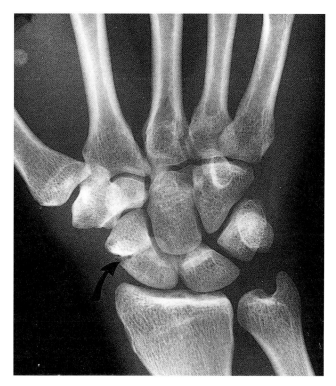

FIG. 30. Scaphoid fracture. PA view of wrist showing minimally displaced fracture through the waist of the scaphoid (*curved arrow*).

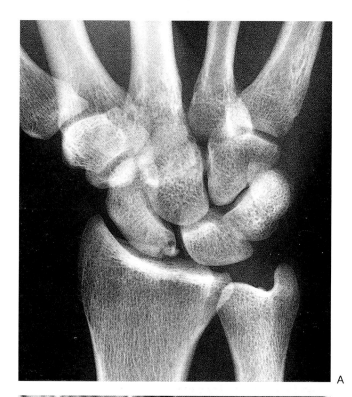

A

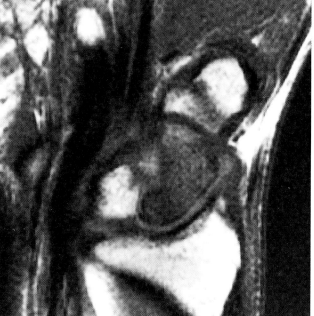

B

FIG. 31. Osteochondral scaphoid fracture. **A:** PA view of wrist in patient who fell on an outstretched hand shows osteochondral fracture of the proximal pole of the scaphoid. **B:** MR image in the same patient shows diffuse, low signal intensity in the navicular compatible with edema, as well as even lower signal intensity in the proximal pole of the scaphoid in the region of the fracture. MR is an exquisitely sensitive test for detecting bone marrow edema.

avascular necrosis (AVN) due to the unique blood supply of this region (49) (Fig. 32). CT is the procedure of choice for evaluating callus formation in suspected nonunion or bone formation after surgical fusion. In cases of nonunion, CT demonstrates a lack of callus bridging the fracture site (22) (Figs. 33 and 34). AVN can be seen as increased sclerosis in the proximal pole after a fracture, but the earliest changes of AVN are best seen with MR imaging (Fig. 35).

Triquetral Fractures

The avulsion fracture of the triquetrum at the attachment of the dorsal radiotriquetral ligament is the second most common carpal fracture in most series (39). This injury has the characteristic appearance of a small fleck of bone seen on the dorsum of the wrist and is best appreciated on the lateral plain film (Fig. 36).

Lunate Fractures

Fracture of the lunate bone accounts for only 3% of carpal fractures (39). It usually is caused by axial compression or hyperextension, and it is represented by volar or dorsal chip fractures, which are very difficult to see on plain films. Although the dorsal chip fracture also may be

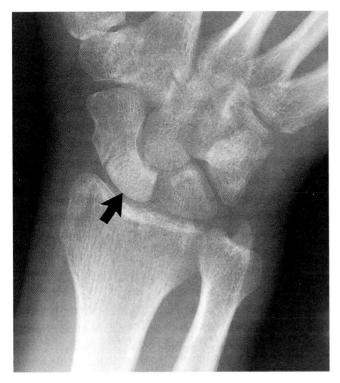

FIG. 32. Scaphoid avascular necrosis (AVN). PA view of wrist in a patient who fell on an outstretched hand 6 weeks before examination. Note the increased sclerosis in the proximal pole of the scaphoid representative of AVN (*arrow*).

difficult to distinguish from the triquetral fracture, this distinction usually is not necessary because both injuries are treated identically with external immobilization (87). In patients with normal plain films and the suspicion of a lunate fracture, CT is the examination of choice to detect this injury (Fig. 37).

There is speculation as to whether lunatomalacia or AVN of the lunate (Kienböck's disease) occurs from trauma because in many cases no acute predisposing traumatic event is found (69). Chronic trauma or stress from compression of the lunate between the capitate and radius, negative ulnar variance with increased axial loading stress on the lunate, and lunate or perilunate dislocation are all thought to predispose to the disease (50,130) (Figs. 38–40).

Hamate Fractures

The hamate bone is protected by its surrounding carpal bones, except for the hamulus, or "hook," which is located on its ventral surface. The hamulus is susceptible to fracture resulting from a fall on the outstretched hand, a sudden forceful blow from a tool handle, or direct impingement by athletic apparatus such as a tennis racket or golf club (23,131). In the acute setting, if a carpal tunnel view cannot be obtained because of pain, an oblique

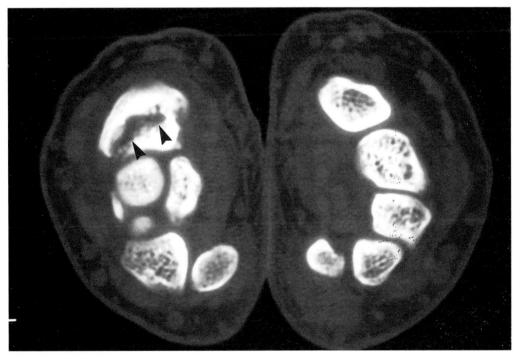

FIG. 33. Nonunion scaphoid fracture. Axial CT image of wrist in patient who had fractured the scaphoid 2 months prior to examination shows a linear lucency through the left scaphoid representing nonunion (*arrowheads*). Direct coronal CT is an alternative projection and may define these fractures to better advantage.

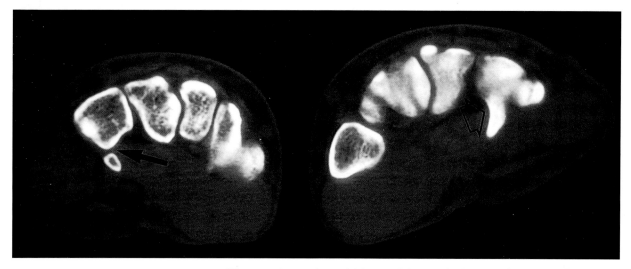

FIG. 34. Hamate nonunion. Axial CT images in a patient with known injury to the hamate show nonunion of the hamate hook fracture (*arrow*). Note the normal hook of the hamate on the contralateral side (*open arrow*).

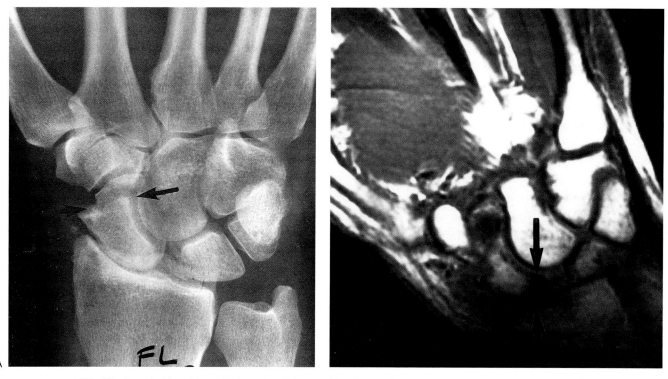

A

B

FIG. 35. Scaphoid AVN on MR imaging. PA plain film (**A**) and T1-weighted coronal MR image (**B**) of the same patient show a fracture of the waist of the scaphoid on the plain film (*arrows*) and low signal intensity within the proximal pole of the scaphoid on MR representing AVN of the proximal pole (*arrows*).

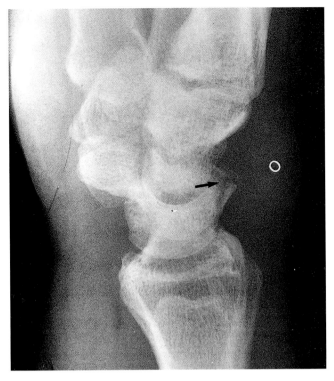

FIG. 36. Triquetral fracture. Lateral view of a patient who fell on an outstretched hand shows a minimally displaced triquetral fracture (*arrow*) with marked soft tissue swelling (○). The lateral view is the best projection for detecting triquetral fractures.

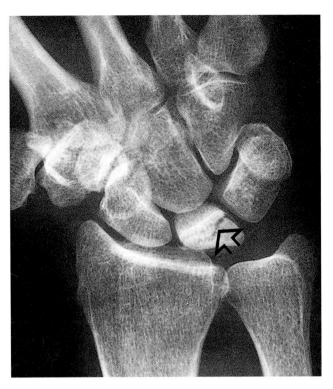

FIG. 38. AVN of the lunate. PA view of wrist in a patient with normal study 3 months prior to this examination shows evidence of AVN of the lunate manifested by increased sclerosis and evidence of a fracture through the midportion of the lunate (*open arrow*).

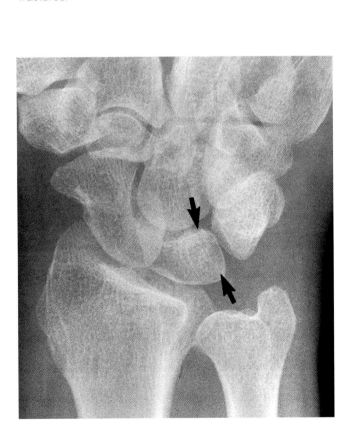

FIG. 37. Lunate fracture. PA view of wrist showing nondisplaced lunate fracture outlined by arrows and arrowhead.

plain film of the forearm in midsupination or of the wrist in minimal dorsiflexion may help to identify the fracture. Lateral tomography and CT are the best imaging tests for diagnosing this injury (41) (see Figs. 19D and 34).

Other Carpal Fractures

Isolated fractures of the pisiform, trapezium, trapezoid, and capitate bones rarely occur from direct blows or falls on the outstretched hand (19). When these cortical injuries cannot be diagnosed on plain films, high-resolution CT best demonstrates them (13,65).

Carpal Dislocations

Trauma with forced dorsiflexion and supination of the carpus on the radius, so that the whole hand "swings round" the medial column of the carpus, is responsible for the majority of carpal dislocations and carpal fracture/dislocations (45). The position of the hand at the time of impact determines the specific abnormality that will be seen (39,45,52,64,136,147,157). Most carpal dislocations are of either the lunate or the perilunate type, with or without associated carpal bone fractures. The or-

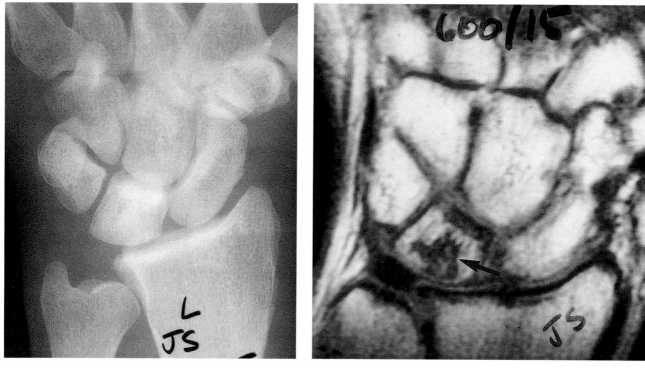

FIG. 39. MR imaging of AVN of the lunate. **A:** PA view of wrist in patient with negative ulnar variance shows increased sclerosis in the lunate compatible with AVN. **B:** T1-weighted coronal MR scan shows an area of low signal intensity in the lunate representing AVN (*arrow*).

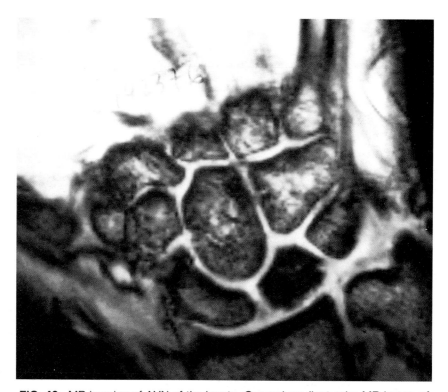

FIG. 40. MR imaging of AVN of the lunate. Coronal gradient echo MR image of patient with plain-film evidence of AVN shows extremely low signal intensity in the region of the lunate compatible with AVN. MR imaging is the best examination for showing early changes of AVN.

thopaedic therapy for either of these is identical in the majority of patients (51,58,85). The key to the diagnosis of each of these patterns is the colinearity of the distal radius, lunate, and capitate, best seen on the lateral view of the wrist.

The distal radial articular surface is the major point of reference in classifying these injuries. With perilunate dislocation, the lunate remains centered over the distal radius, and the remainder of the distal carpal row (best detected by noting the position of the capitate) is displaced volarly (Fig. 41). Perilunate dislocation precedes lunate dislocation (78). With a continued hyperextension force, as may occur with straightening of the hand or with closed manipulation of the perilunate dislocation, the capitate may force the lunate ventrally. When this happens, the lunate is positioned ventrally in relation to the distal radial articular surface, the distal carpal row remains centered over the radius, and "lunate dislocation" is present (Fig. 42). If neither the capitate nor the lunate remains centered over the distal radial articular surface, the term *midcarpal dislocation* is used to identify the pattern (see Fig. 41).

When the injury results in a fracture of one of the carpal bones, the terminology of the injury includes the fractured bone with the prefix *trans-* and the direction of dislocation of the carpal bones (21,44,51,151,152,156). For example, perilunate dislocation in a dorsal direction with a fracture of the scaphoid is referred to as *transscaphoid dorsal perilunate dislocation* (see Figs. 41 and 43).

Carpal Instability

Carpal instability results from weakening (stretching) or disruption of some of the intercarpal ligaments, the radiocarpal ligaments, or both, from bony fracture or from cartilaginous damage (76). With this insult, the carpal bones lose their normal alignment and exhibit abnormal motion. Although these conditions may not be symptomatic, they usually are progressive and may lead to weakness with degenerative change in the wrist, which is a major cause of compensation for loss of hand and wrist function. Carpal instabilities may be static, in which case they can be recognized on the plain films, or dynamic, and therefore can be seen only by fluoroscopic monitoring of the wrist during motion.

The five major types of carpal ligamentous instabilities are listed in Table 3 and shown in Fig. 44 (77). The plain-film diagnosis of these patterns is best made by the "instability series" (139) (Table 4).

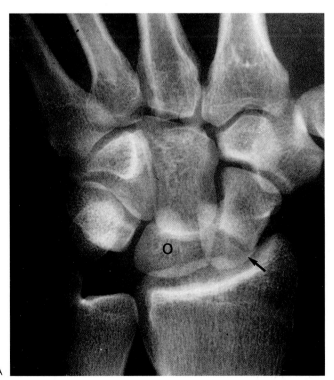 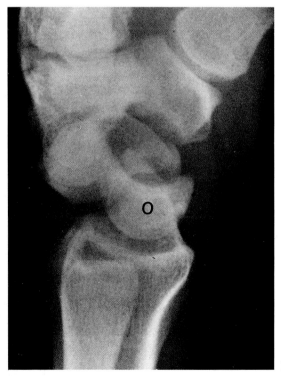

A   B

FIG. 41. Transscaphoid dorsal perilunate dislocation. PA (**A**) and lateral (**B**) views of the wrist showing scaphoid fracture (*arrow*) with dorsal perilunate dislocation, best seen on the lateral projection. Note the position of the lunate in both projections (○).

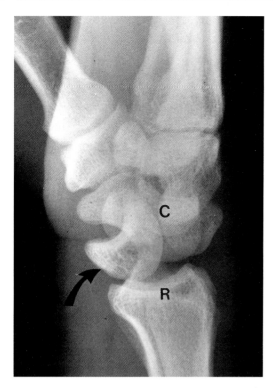

FIG. 42. Lunate dislocation. Lateral view of wrist showing lunate dislocation (*curved arrow*). Note the relatively normal position of the distal radius (R) and capitate (C).

Normal Carpal Relationships

On the neutral lateral film, the central axes of the radial concavity, the lunate concavity, the capitate, and the third metacarpal are essentially colinear (see Fig. 11). However, true colinearity of the distal radius, lunate, and capitate is seen in only 11% of normal wrists (123).

The most important normal relationship in the neutral lateral view is the scapholunate angle, which ranges from 30° to 60° in the normal situation and may be normal up to 80°. The capitolunate angle is normally less than 30° (54,76) (Figs. 12–14).

At fluoroscopy, the carpal bones are visualized in the lateral projection, "flex on flexion," and "extend on extension" (54). The action of the proximal carpal row is best recognized in the lateral projection by the central axis of the lunate, which should flex with respect to the radius on flexion. The capitate (or reference for the distal carpal row) should also be slightly flexed in relation to the lunate axis (Fig. 45). These relationships should be maintained in extension, and both should flex slightly (Fig. 46).

Dorsal Intercalated Segmental Instability (DISI)

DISI is most commonly seen after unstable scaphoid fractures, after radial fractures, secondary to degenera-

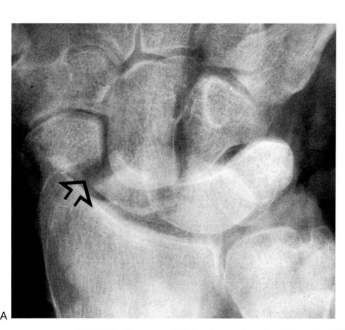

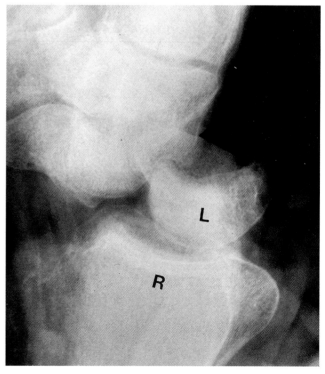

FIG. 43. Transcaphoid volar perilunate dislocation. PA (**A**) and lateral (**B**) views of a severely traumatized wrist showing transcaphoid volar perilunate dislocation. Note the relatively normal relationship of the distal radius (R) and lunate (L) on the lateral film.

TABLE 3. *Ligamentous instability of the wrist*

Ligamentous instability[a]	Scapholunate angle (°)	Capitolunate angle (°)	Comments
Normal	30–60	0–30	—
Dorsiflexion (dorsal when intercalated segmental instability (lateral view): lunate tilts dorsally and scaphoid tilts palmarly	a. 60–80 (?abnormal) b. 80 (abnormal)	Normal or increased	Present when either the scapholunate or the capitolunate angle is abnormal and abnormal intercarpal motion exists
Palmar flexion (ventral intercalated segmental instability) (lateral view): both lunate and scaphoid tilt palmarly	30	30 or normal	
Ulnar translocation (posteroanterior view): carpal bones are ulnar in position	Normal	Normal	Space increased between scaphoid and radial styloid; over 50% of lunate is medial to radius on neutral posteroanterior hand position
Dorsal subluxation (lateral view): carpal bones are dorsal to midplane of the radius	Normal	Normal	
Palmar subluxation (lateral view): carpal bones are palmar to midplane of the radius	Normal	Normal	

From Gilula and Weeks, ref. 54, with permission.

[a] Dorsiflexion, palmar flexion, ulnar translocation, and dorsal carpal subluxation are four not uncommon abnormalities of the wrist. Early detection of these carpal instabilities is necessary in order to obtain effective treatment. Diagnosis depends on *identifying the lunate* and, when necessary, measuring the scapholunate and capitolunate angles.

tive intercarpal arthrosis, and in many cases of scapholunate dissociation. This instability is associated with tears of the volar radiolunotriquetral ligament and the ulnolunate ligament, as well as the intraarticular scapholunate and radioscapholunate ligaments (76,77). In DISI, the scaphoid bone becomes palmar-flexed and the lunate bone faces more dorsally than normal. The result is an increase in the scapholunate angle, which is abnormal if greater than 80°, and an increase in the capitolunate angle to greater than 30° (Fig. 47). DISI also may be secondary to abnormal intercarpal motion without scapholunate diastasis. In this situation, the capitolunate relationship may be normal on the static films, but the instability series may show the DISI patterns, particularly the lateral full flexion and extension, and radial and ulnar deviation views. The results of these examinations are best interpreted by comparing them with the normal

TABLE 4. *Routine radiographic series for instability of the wrist*

PA view with forearm in neutral position
PA view with radial deviation
PA view with ulnar deviation
PA view with tightly clenched fist
Semisupination view
Lateral view with extreme elbow flexion
Lateral view with extreme elbow extension
Lateral view with forearm in neutral position and fist clenched

From Gilula and Weeks, ref. 54, with permission.

side so that subtle abnormal carpal motion may be appreciated (54).

Scapholunate Dissociation

Scapholunate dissociation indicates that the scapholunate ligament has been torn. The classical appearance of this instability is seen on the PA wrist view as a palmar-flexed foreshortened scaphoid bone exhibiting a signet ring sign, a scapholunate gap greater than 4 mm, a dorsiflexed quadrangular lunate, and a dorsiflexed triquetrum that is distal on the hamate (Fig. 48). With marked palmar tilt of the scaphoid from a tear of the ventral radioscapholunate ligament, the scaphoid rotates due to a built-in spring effect and allows the proximal pole to migrate dorsally. The term *rotatory subluxation of the navicular* may be used for this condition (54,139) (Fig. 49). Destabilization of the scaphoid prevents synchronous motion between the proximal and distal carpal rows. On static films, the PA view must not be obtained with radial deviation because this may give a false signet ring sign (see Fig. 7). However, in the false subluxation, the lunate has a triangular shape; in the true subluxation, the lunate is quadrangular.

Volar (Palmar) Intercalated Segmental Instability (VISI)

VISI is the opposite of DISI and is seen after lunotriquetral interosseous ligament disruption, excision of the

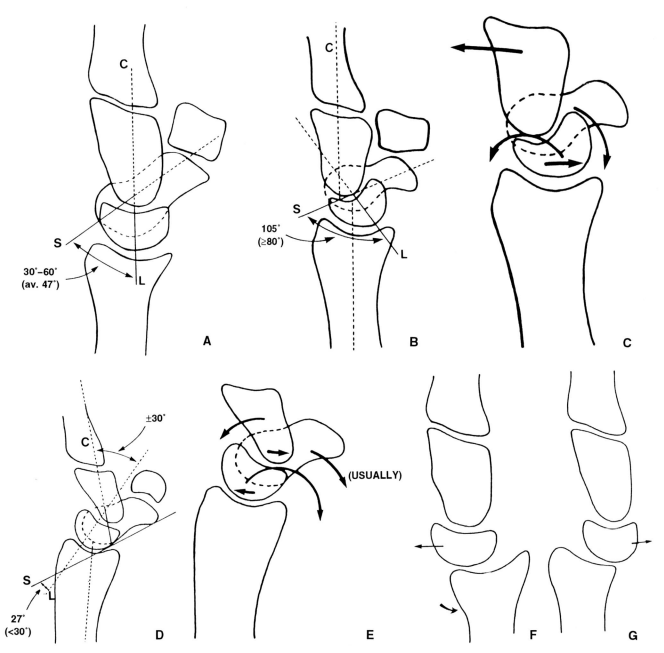

FIG. 44. A: The axes of the capitate (C), lunate (L), and scaphoid (S) bones are represented by the solid and dashed straight lines. A normal scapholunate angle is 30°–60° with an average angle of 47°. The radius, capitate, and lunate axes in this diagram coincide. (Modified from Dobyns et al., AAOS Instructional Course Lectures, 1975, Chapter 11, pp. 182–199, by permission of the authors and publisher.) **B:** Dorsiflexion instability can be diagnosed radiographically when the scapholunate angle is 80° or more. C, capitate; S, scaphoid; L, lunate axes. (Modified from Dobyns et al., ref. 38.) **C:** In dorsiflexion instability the lunate has rotated or tilted so that its distal articular surface faces dorsally, and the capitate is dorsal to the midplane of the radius. The scaphoid (navicular) stays in normal position, or its distal palmar tip moves toward the radius (tilts palmarly or ventrally). Curved arrows show the path of carpal bone rotary motion. The straight arrows indicate the direction of bone movement or displacement. **D:** Palmar flexion instability is diagnosed when the capitolunate angle is 30° or more, or the scapholunate angle is less than 30°. C, capitate; S, scaphoid; L, lunate axes. (Modified from Dobyns et al., ref. 38.) **E:** With palmar flexion instability the distal articular surface of the lunate faces palmarly (ventrally), and the scaphoid usually tilts palmarly with the lunate. The central axis of the capitate lies palmar to the central radial axis, and the capitate may tilt dorsally. The curved arrows represent carpal bone rotation. Straight arrows indicate direction of bone movement or displacement. **F:** Dorsal carpal subluxation exists when all the carpal bones lie dorsal to the center of the distal radial articular surface. The curved arrow indicates an impacted fracture deformity of the distal dorsal radius; the straight arrow indicates dorsal movement of the carpus (carpal bones). **G:** Palmar carpal subluxation would exist when the lunate and other carpal bones lie palmar to the central axis of the radius. The arrow indicates palmar movement of the carpal bones. (From Gilula and Weeks, ref. 54, with permission.)

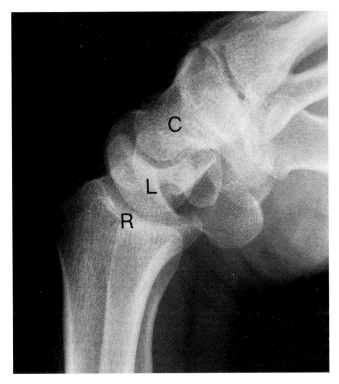

FIG. 45. Normal lateral flexion view of wrist. Lateral flexion view of wrist showing slight flexion of the radius (R), lunate (L), and capitate (C) in the flexed position.

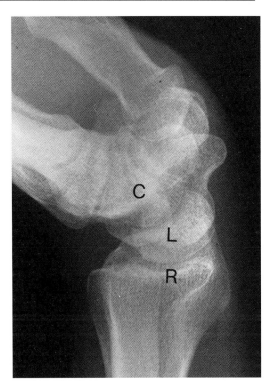

FIG. 46. Normal lateral extension view of wrist. Lateral view of wrist in extension shows slight extension of the lunate (L) and capitate (C) in relation to the radius (R).

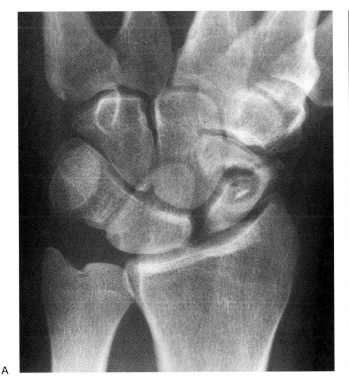

A

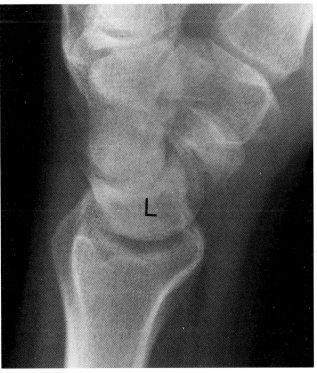

B

FIG. 47. DISI deformity. PA (**A**) and lateral (**B**) views of the wrist in patient with scaphoid fracture non-union shows dorsal tilt of the lunate (L) on the lateral view, representing the DISI deformity.

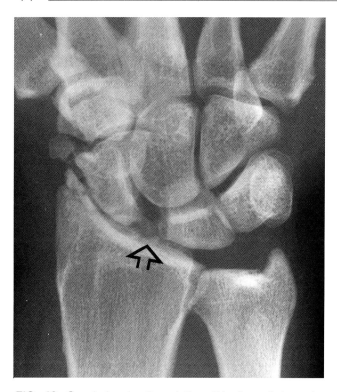

FIG. 48. Scapholunate dissociation. PA view of the wrist showing healed fracture of the distal radius and ulnar styloid with marked widening at the scapholunate junction, representing scapholunate dissociation (*open arrow*).

triquetrum, sprains of the midcarpal joint that attenuate extrinsic ligaments, or, rarely, as a normal variant in people with lax ligamentous structures (77).

The traumatic version of VISI is lunotriquetral dissociation (L-T dissociation). In this instability, the PA wrist view shows a palmar-flexed foreshortened scaphoid bone, but there is no widening of the scapholunate gap. The lunate may tilt palmarly more than the scaphoid so that there is a break in the normal arc of the proximal carpal row on the PA view, and the angle as measured on the lateral view is less than 30°. The capitate head moves anteriorly while its distal aspect moves dorsally, and the capitolunate angle increases to over 30°. This condition also may be found in asymptomatic patients (54) (Fig. 50).

Ulnar Translocation

Ulnar translocation instability, a rare situation most commonly seen after trauma or in rheumatoid arthritis, is caused by tearing of the ventral and dorsal radiolunate and radiocapitate ligaments. Absence of these strong ligaments permits ulnar subluxation of the carpus. It is best determined on the PA view when a gap develops between the radial styloid and the lateral scaphoid border, when the scaphoid is not centered over the distal radial con-

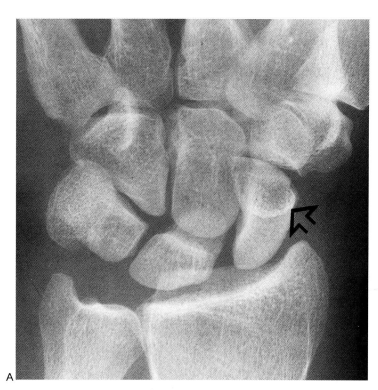

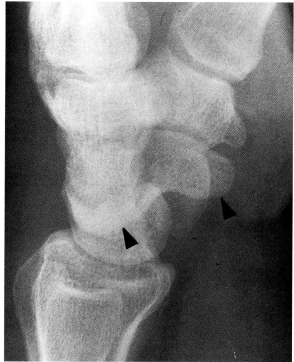

FIG. 49. Rotatory subluxation of the scaphoid. PA (**A**) and lateral (**B**) views of the wrist in a patient who had fallen on the outstretched hand shows the signet ring appearance of the scaphoid on the PA view (*open arrow*) and the palmar tilt of the scaphoid on the lateral view (*arrowheads*) representing rotatory subluxation.

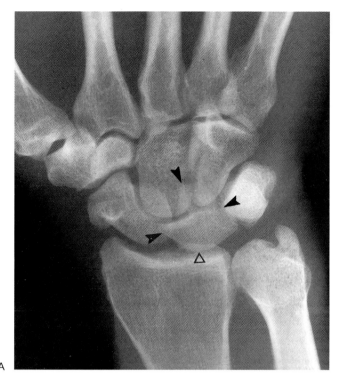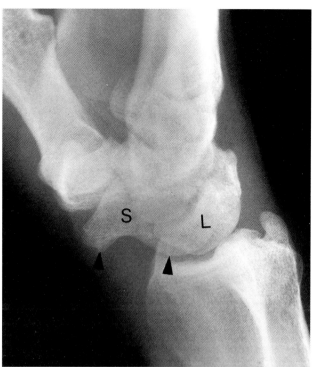

A　　　　　　　　　　　　　　　　　　　　　　　　　　　　　B

FIG. 50. VISI deformity. PA (**A**) and lateral (**B**) views of the wrist in a patient showing the VISI deformity. Note the triangular shape of the lunate (*arrowheads*), the break in the proximal carpal arc with proximal displacement of the lunate (*open arrowhead*), and the palmar tilt of the lunate (L) on the lateral film, with marked decrease in the scapholunate angle to less than 30°. S, scaphoid.

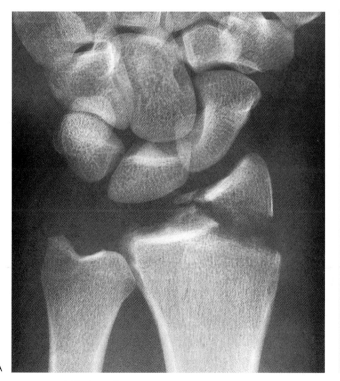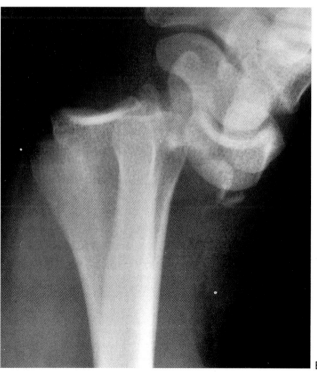

A　　　　　　　　　　　　　　　　　　　　　　　　　　　　　B

FIG. 51. Dorsal carpal subluxation. PA (**A**) and lateral (**B**) views of the wrist in a patient after significant trauma shows intraarticular fracture of the distal radius with dorsal subluxation of the carpus best seen on the lateral film. Note the widening at the radiocarpal junction on the PA view.

cavity, when the trapezium (greater multangular) closely abuts the radial styloid, or when over 50% of the lunate lies medial to the distal radius (54,77).

Dorsal Palmar Carpal Subluxation

Dorsal subluxation of the carpus is rare. Most commonly it is seen after a severely impacted Colle's fracture (38,52,54). In this instability pattern, the lateral film demonstrates that the lunate is displaced and is no longer centered over the radial articular surface (Fig. 51). The rare palmar carpal subluxation shows scapholunate diastasis, ulnar styloid fractures, and volar radial fractures on the PA view. In the reported cases of this deformity, ulnar translocation also has been present (8).

PATHOLOGIC CONDITIONS OF THE DISTAL RADIOULNAR JOINT

The normal bony relationship of the distal radius and ulna on the plain film is described in the section on normal plain-film anatomy. Pathologic conditions affecting the DRUJ can be divided into acute fractures, osseous nonunion or malunion, RUJ incongruity, and abnormalities of the TFCC (102). Acute fractures are discussed in Chapter 10 on distal radial fractures.

DRUJ Subluxation/Dislocation/Diastasis

Gross DRUJ dislocation or diastasis is not usually a difficult diagnostic dilemma. However, diagnosis of DRUJ subluxation may be difficult with plain radiography due to minor degrees of pronation and supination, which may affect interpretation, and to the ulnar and radial movements during these motions (94) (Fig. 52). In most cases of suspected subluxation, CT or MR imaging should be used for definitive diagnosis. At the present time, however, CT is the recommended procedure of the two for evaluation of this articulation due to its lower cost and its superior ability to show the articulation (13,14,20,70,93,94,124,149).

CT criteria for DRUJ subluxation were first defined by Mino and colleagues in 1983 (94). They described parallel lines drawn through the dorsal and palmar borders of the radius in which the ulna resided when the joint was normal. Displacement of the ulna beyond these lines was considered subluxation. However, these criteria are difficult to use because with supination and pronation of the radius there is translation of the relatively fixed ulna so that it lies somewhat palmar in supination and dorsal in pronation (27,70). Therefore, the parallel line method of Mino applies only if the subluxation occurs in the neutral position. Weschler and colleagues further defined the methods of determining DRUJ subluxation (149). Ac-

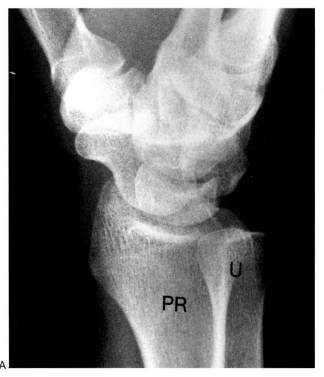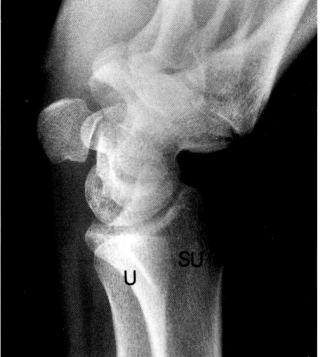

FIG. 52. Semisupination/semipronation views of wrist. **A:** Semipronated view of the wrist showing the relationship of the ulna to the radius. A false diagnosis of radioulnar dislocation will be made if this semipronated positioning is not recognized. **B:** Semisupination lateral view of the wrist showing the inferior positioning of the ulna, which should not be misinterpreted as radioulnar dislocation. U, ulna; SU, semisupinated; PR, semipronated.

cording to the congruity method, the arcs made by the ulnar head and the sigmoid notch should be symmetric in the normal situation. The epicenter method is defined by drawing a perpendicular line from the center of rotation in the distal radioulnar joint to the cord of the sigmoid notch: If the line is in the middle half of the sigmoid notch, it is considered normal. A third method, the radioulnar line method, defines the radius as normal if the head falls between two lines drawn on each side of the ulna (Figs. 53 and 54). Subluxation may occur in only one position. King and colleagues have shown that palmar subluxation of the ulna is best shown with the pronation scan and that dorsal subluxation and radioulnar diastasis are best detected by the neutral scan (70). Therefore, for adequate evaluation of DRUJ subluxation, thin (5 mm) contiguous CT sections should be obtained through the joint in the supinated, neutral, and pronated positions, using the above criteria. MR imaging is an alternative imaging test to determine radioulnar dislocation (Fig. 55).

Ulnar Variance

Ulnar variance refers to the relative lengths of the radius and ulna as visualized at their articulation with the lunate on the correctly positioned AP wrist radiograph. Abnormalities may be congenital, or they may be secondary to trauma or surgery.

Adequate assessment of ulnar variance requires that the PA wrist films be obtained with the elbow flexed to 90°, the shoulder abducted to 90°, and the forearm in neutral rotation with the wrist in ulnar deviation, as this position shows clear ulnar and lunate landmarks (43,60). It should be remembered that ulnar variance is dependent on position and grip during the radiographic examination. Maximal forearm pronation and powerful grip lengthen the ulna relative to the radius, and maximal supination relatively decreases ulnar length. These measurements may change as much as 1–2 mm, depending on the examination technique (43,105).

"Negative ulnar variance," or a short ulna relative to the radius, is seen more often in AVN or malacia of the lunate (Kienböck's disease), due to the heightened axial loading borne by the lunate with this abnormal distal radioulnar relationship (50,67,105,108). Kienböck's disease can be staged according to radiographic criteria (2):

Stage I: Normal lunate contour; evidence of compression fracture
Stage II: Bony resorption along fracture
Stage III: Stage I and II changes with bony sclerosis
Stage IV: Flattening and fragmentation of lunate
Stage V: Radiocarpal joint arthrosis

Plain films, bone scans, conventional tomography, and CT can detect the consequences of Kienböck's disease. However, MR imaging is the only technique that adequately assesses the integrity of the fatty marrow within the lunate and directly images the articular cartilage destruction and accompanying synovitis of the late stages of the disease (116). Therefore, in the suspected

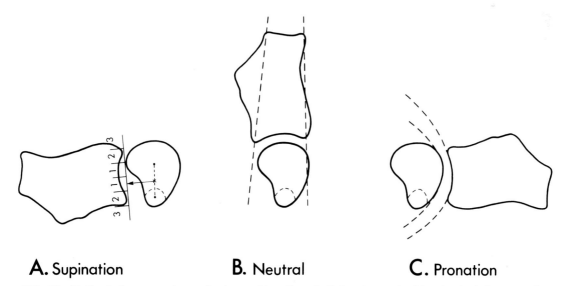

A. Supination   **B.** Neutral   **C.** Pronation

FIG. 53. Methods for assessing radioulnar subluxation. **A:** Epicenter method (supination). A perpendicular line is drawn from the center of rotation of the distal radioulnar joint (a point halfway between the ulnar styloid process and center of the ulnar head) to the cord of the sigmoid notch. It is considered normal if this line is in the middle half of the sigmoid notch. (*Dotted lines* represent the location of the styloid process, which in many cases is extrapolated from contiguous distal scans.) **B:** Radioulnar line method (neutral). Articulation of the ulnar head with the radius is normal if the head falls between the two lines pictured above. **C:** Congruity method (pronation). Note congruity of the arc of the ulnar head with that of the sigmoid notch. (From Wechsler, ref. 149, with permission.)

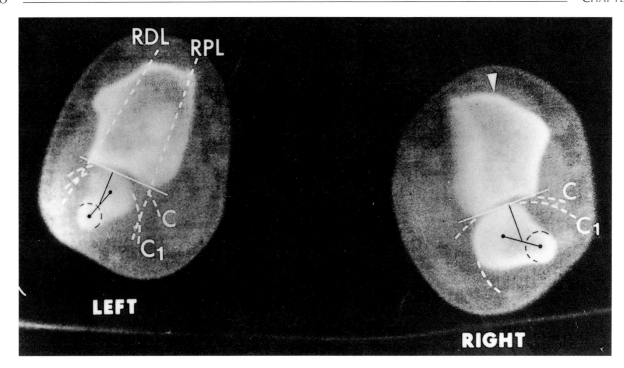

FIG. 54. Normal left wrist (neutral position) by all three criteria. Rounded aspect (*arrowhead*) of the lateral aspect of the distal right radius makes the use of the radioulnar lines difficult. The other two methods reveal no evidence of radioulnar subluxation. C, arc of the sigmoid notch; C_1, arc of the ulnar head; RDL, radioulnar line; RPL, radiopalmar line. (From Wechsler, ref. 149, with permission.)

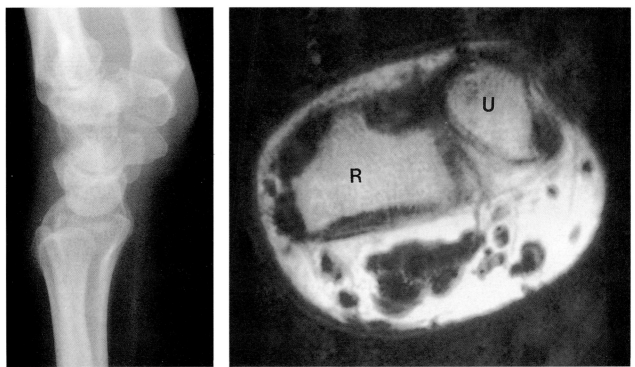

A   B

FIG. 55. Radioulnar dislocation. Neutral lateral plain film (**A**) and axial T1-weighted MR scan (**B**) in patient after trauma shows superior displacement of the ulna in relation to the radius, representing radioulnar dislocation.

early stages of Kienböck's disease, MR imaging is the preferred imaging modality (see Figs. 38 and 39).

Positive ulnar variance, or a long ulna relative to the radius, predisposes to the ulnocarpal impaction syndrome and perforations of the TFCC (15,36,48,91, 104,105) (Fig. 56). The diagnosis of the ulnocarpal impaction syndrome is made most often on clinical grounds, although radiographs of the wrist may show positive ulnar variance, malunion of a distal radial fracture with residual radial shortening and abnormal dorsal tilt, postsurgical altering of the normal radioulnar relationship, or secondary changes of subchondral sclerosis and cystic regions in the lunate or ulnar head (Fig. 57). Arthrography in these cases may show rupture of the lunotriquetral ligament or the TFCC (48).

TFCC Abnormalities

Abnormalities of the TFCC, the meniscal homologue of the wrist, are usually caused by trauma or degeneration. Tears of the TFCC are age-related; few perforations are recognized in anatomic dissections before the fourth decade (145). The incidence of TFCC tears increases with age, and by the sixth decade over 50% of cadaveric specimens demonstrate perforations (91,105). Rupture

of the lunotriquetral ligament may also be seen in up to 75% of patients with TFCC tears (105,145). The association of positive ulnar variance and TFCC perforations is further proved by data showing that 73% of neutral or positive ulnar variance specimens have TFCC tears, whereas only 17% of wrists with negative ulnar variance exhibit this finding (105). In fact, some authors believe that all TFCC perforations with negative ulnar variance are traumatic in origin (57).

Before the availability of MR imaging, tears of the TFCC were diagnosed best by arthrography (35,96). Injection of contrast material into the DRUJ can show perforations through the TFCC with contrast extending into the DRUJ (see Fig. 26B). Because some TFCC perforations are reported to have one-way valve-like compartmental communications, some authors recommend injecting contrast medium into the DRUJ as well in order to exclude these tears (74).

MR imaging, however, now offers a noninvasive, highly accurate alternative to arthrography in the diagnosis of TFCC tears (33,55). Tears are recognized on MR imaging as linear areas of increased signal intensity through the normally low-signal-intensity TFCC on both T1-weighted and T2-weighted images. Fluid also may be present in the adjacent wrist compartments (Fig.

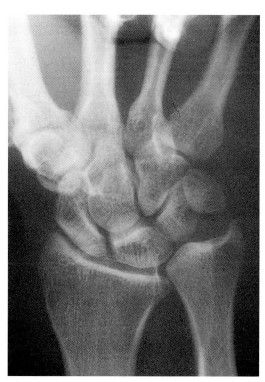

FIG. 56. Positive ulnar variance. PA view of the wrist showing marked positive ulnar variance, which in this patient was a congenital abnormality. The most common cause is distal radial fractures. This deformity predisposes to tears of the TFCC.

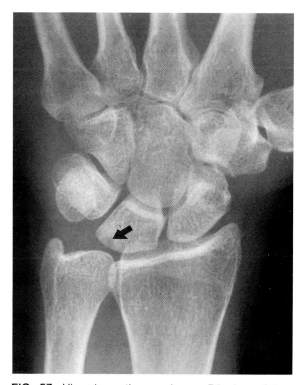

FIG. 57. Ulnar impaction syndrome. PA view of the wrist showing positive ulnar variance and cystic change in the lunate characteristic of ulnar impaction syndrome (arrow).

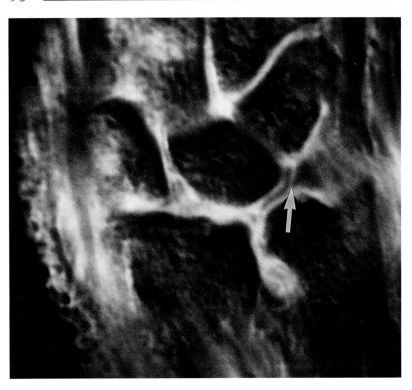

FIG. 58. TFCC tear by MR imaging. Coronal gradient echo image of MR scan of the wrist shows a linear area with high signal intensity through the TFCC representing an arthroscopically proven TFCC tear (*white arrow*).

58). TFCC tears occur near the radial insertion in some series and near the ulnar insertion in others; there is excellent correlation with arthrography (55,159). In fact, some authors believe that TFCC degeneration occurring before perforation (similar to meniscal degeneration) may be seen on MR imaging as areas of increased signal intensity within the TFCC that do not communicate with the articular surface. These observations need follow-up confirmation (59).

Dedicated "small parts" coils and fast spin-echo techniques will undoubtedly increase the potential of MR imaging for diagnosing TFCC and ligamentous abnormalities. However, at the present time, both arthrography and MR imaging are acceptable techniques to use in evaluating the TFCC.

In summary, this chapter briefly describes the tests available in the imaging evaluation of the wrist and suggests an algorithmic approach to diagnosis in this complex anatomic region.

ACKNOWLEDGMENTS

I appreciate the excellent administrative assistance of Angela Overby, Donna Garrison, and Nancy Ragland. The technical assistance of John Cassell, Dennis Daniels, and Rita Lee is also greatly appreciated.

REFERENCES

1. Abbitt PL, Riddervold HO. The carpal tunnel view: Helpful adjuvant for unrecognized fractures of the carpus. *Skeletal Radiol* 1987;16:45–47.
2. Almquist EA. Kienböck's disease. *Hand Clin* 1987;3:141–148.
3. Amadio PC, Berquist TH, Smith DK, Ilstrup DM, Cooney WP III, Linscheid RL. Scaphoid malunion. *J Hand Surg* 1989;14A: 679–687.
4. Amadio PC, Hanssen AD, Berquist TH. The genesis of Kienböck's disease: Evaluation of a case by magnetic resonance imaging. *J Hand Surg* 1987;12A:1044–1049.
5. Arkless R. Cineradiography in normal and abnormal wrists. *AJR* 1966;96:837–844.
6. Baker LL, Hajek PC, Bjorkengren A, et al. High-resolution magnetic resonance imaging of the wrist: Normal anatomy. *Skeletal Radiol* 1987;16:128–132.
7. Ballinger PW. *Merrill's Atlas of Radiographic Positions and Radiologic Procedures,* Vols. 1–3. 7th Ed. St. Louis: Mosby-Yearbook, 1991.
8. Bellinghausen H-W, Gilula LA, Young LV, Weeks PM. Posttraumatic palmar carpal subluxation. Report of two patients. *J Bone Joint Surg* 1983;65A:998–1006.
9. Belsole RJ, Hilbelink D, Llewellyn JA, Dale M, Stenzler S, Rayhack JM. Scaphoid orientation and location from computed, three-dimensional carpal models. *Orthop Clin North Am* 1986;17:505–510.
10. Belsole RJ, Hilbelink DR, Llewellyn JA, Stenzler S, Greene TL, Dale M. Mathematical analysis of computed carpal models. *J Orthop Res* 1988;6:116–122.
11. Binkovitz LA, Berquist TH, McLeod RA. Masses of the hand and wrist: Detection and characterization with MR imaging. *AJR* 1990;154:323–326.
12. Binkovitz LA, Ehman RL, Cahill DR, Berquist TH. Magnetic resonance imaging of the wrist: Normal cross sectional imaging and selected abnormal cases. *Radiographics* 1988;8:1171–1202.
13. Biondetti PR, Vannier MW, Gilula LA, Knapp R. Wrist: Coronal and transaxial CT scanning. *Radiology* 1987;163:149–151.
14. Bowers WH. Instability of the distal radioulnar articulation. *Hand Clin* 1991;7:311–327.
15. Bowers WH. The distal radioulnar joint. In: Green DP, ed. *Operative Hand Surgery.* Vol. 2. 2nd Ed. New York: Churchill Livingstone, 1988, pp. 939–989.
16. Boyes JM. More accurate diagnosis of hand and wrist injuries. *Consultant* 1973;56:1459.
17. Braunstein EM, Louis DS, Greene TL, Hankin FM. Fluoroscopic

and arthrographic evaluation of carpal instability. *AJR* 1985;144:1259–1262.
18. Bresina SJ, Vannier MW, Logan SE, Weeks PM. Three-dimensional wrist imaging: Evaluation of functional and pathologic anatomy by computer. *Clin Plast Surg* 1986;13:389–405.
19. Bryan RS, Dobyns JH. Fractures of the carpal bones other than lunate and navicular. *Clin Orthop* 1980;149:107–111.
20. Burk DL Jr, Karasick D, Wechsler RJ. Imaging of the distal radioulnar joint. *Hand Clin* 1991;7:263–275.
21. Burman MS, Sinberg SE, Gersh W, Schmier AA. Fractures of the radial and ulnar axes. A unifying concept, with a description of certain carpal injuries, including parallel and gear rotations of the carpal bones. *AJR* 1944;51:455–480.
22. Bush CH, Gillespy T III, Dell PC. High-resolution CT of the wrist: Initial experience with scaphoid disorders and surgical fusions. *AJR* 1987;149:757–760.
23. Carter PR, Eaton RG, Littler JW. Ununited fracture of the hook of the hamate. *J Bone Joint Surg* 1977;59A:583–588.
24. Carver RA, Barrington NA. Soft-tissue changes accompanying recent scaphoid injuries. *Clin Radiol* 1985;36:423–425.
25. Cerofolini E, Luchetti R, Pederzini L, et al. MR evaluation of triangular fibrocartilage complex tears in the wrist: Comparison with arthrography and arthroscopy. *J Comput Assist Tomogr* 1990;14:963–967.
26. Clark KC. *Positioning in Radiography.* Vol. 1. 9th Ed. Chicago: Yearbook, 1973.
27. Cone RO, Szabo R, Resnick D, Gelberman R, Taleisnik J, Gilula LA. Computed tomography of the normal radioulnar joints. *Invest Radiol* 1983;18:541–545.
28. Conway WF, Hayes CW. Three-compartment wrist arthrography: Use of a low-iodine-concentration contrast agent to decrease study time. *Radiology* 1989;173:569–570.
29. Cooney WP, Linscheid RL, Dobyns JH. Scaphoid fractures. Problems associated with nonunion and avascular necrosis. *Orthop Clin North Am* 1984;15:381–391.
30. Crittenden JJ, Jones DM, Santarelli AG. Bilateral rotational dislocation of the carpal navicular. *Radiology* 1970;94:629–630.
31. Curtis DJ. Injuries of the wrist: an approach to diagnosis. *Radiol Clin North Am* 1981;19:625–644.
32. Curtis DJ, Downey EF Jr, Brower AC, Cruess DF, Herrington WT, Ghaed N. Importance of soft-tissue evaluation in hand and wrist trauma: Statistical evaluation. *AJR* 1984;142:781–788.
33. Dalinka MK, Meyer S, Kricun ME, Vanel D. Magnetic resonance imaging of the wrist. *Hand Clin* 1991;7:87–98.
34. Dalinka MK, Osterman AL, Albert AS, Harty M. Arthrography of the wrist and shoulder. *Orthop Clin North Am* 1983;14(1):193–215.
35. Dalinka MK, Turner ML, Osterman DL, Batra P. Wrist arthrography. *Radiol Clin North Am* 1981;19:217–226.
36. Darrow JC Jr, Linscheid RL, Dobyns JH, Mann JM III, Wood MB, Beckenbaugh RD. Distal ulnar recession for disorders of the distal radioulnar joint. *J Hand Surg* 1985;10A:482–491.
37. Desser TS, McCarthy S, Trumble T. Scaphoid fractures and Kienböck's disease of the lunate: MR imaging with histopathologic correlation. *Magn Reson Imaging* 1990;8:357–361.
38. Dobyns JH, Linscheid RL. Fractures and dislocations of the wrist. In: Rockwood CA Jr, Green DP, eds. *Fractures.* Vol. 1. Philadelphia: JB Lippincott, 1975; pp. 345–440.
39. Dunn AW. Fractures and dislocations of the carpus. *Surg Clin North Am* 1972;52:1513–1538.
40. Duszynski DO, Kuhn JP, Afshani E, Riddlesberger MM Jr. Early radionuclide diagnosis of acute osteomyelitis. *Radiology* 1975;117:337–340.
41. Egawa M, Asai T. Fracture of the hook of the hamate: report of six cases and the suitability of computerized tomography. *J Hand Surg* 1983;8A:393–398.
42. Engel J, Salai M, Yaffe B, Tadmor R. The role of three dimension computerized imaging in hand surgery. *J Hand Surg* 1987;12B:349–352.
43. Epner RA, Bowers WH, Guilford WB. Ulnar variance—the effect of wrist positioning and roentgen filming technique. *J Hand Surg* 1982;7A:298–305.
44. Fisk GR. Carpal instability and the fractured scaphoid. *Ann R Coll Surg Engl* 1970;46:63–76.
45. Fisk GR. The wrist. *J Bone Joint Surg* 1984;66B:396–407.
46. Fornage BD, Schernberg FL, Rifkin MD. Ultrasound examination of the hand. *Radiology* 1985;155:785–788.
47. Frahm R, Saul O, Mannerfelt L. Diagnostic applications of wrist arthrography. *Arch Orthop Trauma Surg* 1990;109:39–42.
48. Friedman SL, Palmer AK. The ulnar impaction syndrome. *Hand Clin* 1991;7:295–310.
49. Gelberman RH, Gross MS. The vascularity of the wrist. Identification of arterial patterns at risk. *Clin Orthop* 1986;202:40–49.
50. Gelberman RH, Salamon PB, Jurist JM, Posch JL. Ulnar variance in Kienböck's disease. *J Bone Joint Surg* 1975;57A:674–676.
51. Gilula LA. Carpal injuries: Analytic approach and case exercises. *AJR* 1979;133:503–517.
52. Gilula LA, Destouet JM, Weeks PM, Young LV, Wray RC. Roentgenographic diagnosis of the painful wrist. *Clin Orthop* 1984;187:52–64.
53. Gilula LA, Totty WG, Weeks PM. Wrist arthrography. The value of fluoroscopic spot viewing. *Radiology* 1983;146:555–556.
54. Gilula LA, Weeks PM. Post-traumatic ligamentous instabilities of the wrist. *Radiology* 1978;129:641–651.
55. Golimbu CN, Firooznia H, Melone CP Jr, Rafii M, Weinreb J, Leber C. Tears of the triangular fibrocartilage of the wrist: MR imaging. *Radiology* 1989;173:731–733.
56. Graziani A. L'esame radiologic del carpo. *Radiol Med* 1940;27:382–392.
57. Greenan T, Zlatkin MB. Magnetic resonance imaging of the wrist. *Semin Ultrasound CT MR* 1990;11:267–287.
58. Green DP, O'Brien ET. Open reduction of carpal dislocations: Indications and operative techniques. *J Hand Surg* 1978;3A:250–265.
59. Gundry CR, Kursunoglu-Brahme S, Schwaighofer B, Kang HS, Sartoris DJ, Resnick D. Is MR better than arthrography for evaluating the ligaments of the wrist? In vitro study. *AJR* 1990;154:337–341.
60. Hardy DC, Totty WG, Reinus WR, Gilula LA. Posteroanterior wrist radiography: Importance of arm positioning. *J Hand Surg* 1987;12A:504–508.
61. Hart VL, Gaynor V. Roentgenographic study of the carpal canal. *J Bone Joint Surg* 1941;23A:382–383.
62. Herbert TJ, Faithfull RG, McCann DJ, Ireland J. Bilateral arthrography of the wrist. *J Hand Surg* 1990;15B:233–235.
63. Hermann G, Rose JS. Computed tomography in bone and soft tissue pathology of the extremities. *J Comput Assist Tomogr* 1979;3:58–66.
64. Hill NA. Fractures and dislocations of the carpus. *Orthop Clin North Am* 1970;1:275–284.
65. Hindman BW, Kulik WJ, Lee G, Avolio RE. Occult fractures of the carpals and metacarpals: demonstration by CT. *AJR* 1989;153:529–532.
66. Hudson TM, Caragol WJ, Kaye JJ. Isolated rotatory subluxation of the carpal navicular. *AJR* 1976;126:601–611.
67. Hultén O. Uber anatomische Variationen der Handgelenkknochen. *Acta Radiol* 1928;9:155–168.
68. Jeffrey RB Jr, Laing FC, Schechter WP, Markison RE, Barton RM. Acute suppurative tenosynovitis of the hand: Diagnosis with US. *Radiology* 1987;162:741–742.
69. Kienböck R. Concerning traumatic malacia of the lunate and its consequences: degeneration and compression fractures (as translated by L. Peltier). *Clin Orthop* 1980;149:4–8.
70. King GJ, McMurtry RY, Rubenstein JD, Ogston NG. Computerized tomography of the distal radioulnar joint: correlation with ligamentous pathology in a cadaveric model. *J Hand Surg* 1986;11A:711–717.
71. Koenig H, Lucas D, Meissner R. The wrist: A preliminary report on high-resolution MR imaging. *Radiology* 1986;160:463–467.
72. Kursunoglu-Brahme S, Gundry CR, Resnick D. Advanced imaging of the wrist. *Radiol Clin North Am* 1990;28:307–320.
73. Levinsohn EM, Palmer AK. Arthrography of the traumatized wrist. *Radiology* 1983;146:647–651.
74. Levinsohn EM, Palmer AK, Coren AB, Zinberry E. Wrist arthrography: The value of the three compartment injection technique. *Skeletal Radiol* 1987;16:539–544.
75. Levinsohn EM, Rosen ID, Palmer AK. Wrist arthrography: Value of the three-compartment injection method. *Radiology* 1991;179:231–239.

76. Linscheid RL, Dobyns JH, Beabout JW, Bryan RS. Traumatic instability of the wrist. Diagnosis, classification, and pathomechanics. *J Bone Joint Surg* 1972;54A:1612–1632.

77. Linscheid RL, Dobyns JH, Beckenbaugh RD, Cooney WP III, Wood MB. Instability patterns of the wrist. *J Hand Surg* 1983;8A:682–686.

78. MacAusland WR. Perilunar dislocation of the carpal bones and dislocation of the lunate bone. *Surg Gynecol Obstet* 1944;79:256–266.

79. MacKinnon SE, Holder LE. The use of three-phase radionuclide bone scanning in the diagnosis of reflex sympathetic dystrophy. *J Hand Surg* 1984;9A:556–563.

80. Manaster BJ. Digital wrist arthrography: Precision in determining the site of radiocarpal-midcarpal communication. *AJR* 1986;147:563–566.

81. Manaster BJ. The clinical efficacy of triple-injection wrist arthrography. *Radiology* 1991;178:267–270.

82. Manzione N, Pizzutillo PD. Stress fracture of the scaphoid wrist. A case report. *Am J Sports Med* 1981;9:268–269.

83. Martin JR. The role of nuclear medicine bone scans in evaluating pain in athletic injuries. *Clin Sports Med* 1987;6:713–737.

84. Matin P. Bone scintigraphy in the diagnosis and management of traumatic injury. *Semin Nucl Med* 1983;13:104–122.

85. Mayfield JK, Johnson RP, Kilcoyne RK. Carpal dislocations: pathomechanics and progressive perilunar instability. *J Hand Surg* 1980;5A:226–241.

86. Mesgarzadeh M, Schneck CD, Bonakdarpour A, Mitra A, Conaway D. Carpal tunnel: MR imaging. II. Carpal tunnel syndrome. *Radiology* 1989;171:749–754.

87. Meyer S. Radiographic evaluation of wrist trauma. *Semin Roentgenol* 1991;26:300–317.

88. Micheli LJ, Jupiter J. Osteoid osteoma as a cause of knee pain in the young athlete. *Am J Sports Med* 1978;6:199–203.

89. Middleton WD, Kneeland JB, Kellman GM, et al. MR imaging of the carpal tunnel: Normal anatomy and preliminary findings in the carpal tunnel syndrome. *AJR* 1987;148:307–316.

90. Middleton WD, Macrander S, Lawson TL, et al. High resolution surface coil magnetic resonance imaging of the joints: Anatomic correlation. *Radiographics* 1987;7:645–683.

91. Mikic ZD. Age changes in the triangular fibrocartilage of the wrist joint. *J Anat* 1978;126:367–384.

92. Mikic ZD. Arthrography of the wrist joint. An experimental study. *J Bone Joint Surg* 1984;66A:371–378.

93. Mino DE, Palmer AK, Levinsohn EM. Radiography and computerized tomography in the diagnosis of incongruity of the distal radio-ulnar joint. A prospective study. *J Bone Joint Surg* 1985;67A:247–252.

94. Mino DE, Palmer AK, Levinsohn EM. The role of radiography and computerized tomography in the diagnosis of subluxation and dislocation of the distal radioulnar joint. *J Hand Surg* 1983;8A:23–31.

95. Moneim MS. The tangential posteroanterior radiograph to demonstrate scapholunate dissociation. *J Bone Joint Surg* 1981;63A:1324–1326.

96. Mrose HE, Rosenthal DI. Arthrography of the hand and wrist. *Hand Clin* 1991;7:201–217.

97. Mutoh Y, Mori T, Suzuki Y, Sugiura Y. Stress fractures of the ulna in athletes. *Am J Sports Med* 1982;10:365–367.

98. Nakamura R, Horii M, Tanaka T, Imaeda T, Hayakawa N. Three-dimensional CT imaging for wrist disorders. *J Hand Surg* 1989;14B:53–59.

99. Nesbit D, Levine E, Neff JR. Direct longitudinal computed tomography of the forearm. *J Comput Assist Tomogr* 1981;5:144–146.

100. Newberg AH, Wetzner SM. Digital subtraction arthrography. *Radiology* 1985;154:238–239.

101. Norman A, Nelson J, Green S. Fractures of the hook of hamate: radiographic signs. *Radiology* 1985;154:49–53.

102. Palmer AK. The distal radioulnar joint. *Orthop Clin North Am* 1984;15:321–335.

103. Palmer AK, Levinsohn EM, Kuzma GR. Arthrography of the wrist. *J Hand Surg* 1983;8A:15–23.

104. Palmer AK, Werner FW. Biomechanics of the distal radioulnar joint. *Clin Orthop* 1984;187:26–35.

105. Palmer AK, Werner FW. The triangular fibrocartilage complex of the wrist—anatomy and function. *J Hand Surg* 1981;6A:153–162.

106. Patel RB. Evaluation of complex carpal trauma: Thin-section direct longitudinal computed tomography scanning through a plaster cast. *J Comput Tomogr* 1985;9:107–109.

107. Pennes DR, Jonsson K, Buckwalter KA. Direct coronal CT of the scaphoid bone. *Radiology* 1989;171:870–871.

108. Persson M. Causal treatment of lunatomalacia: Further experiences of operative ulna lengthening. *Acta Chir Scand* 1950;100:531–544.

109. Pirela-Cruz MA, Goll SR, Klug M, Windler D. Stress computed tomography analysis of the distal radioulnar joint: A diagnostic tool for determining translational motion. *J Hand Surg* 1991;16A:75–82.

110. Pittman CC, Quinn SF, Belsole R, Greene T, Rayhack J. Digital subtraction wrist arthrography: Use of a double contrast technique as a supplement to single contrast arthrography. *Skeletal Radiol* 1988;17:119–122.

111. Protas JM, Jackson WT. Evaluating carpal instabilities with fluoroscopy. *AJR* 1980;135:137–140.

112. Quinn SF, Belsole RJ, Greene TL, Rayhack JM. Advanced imaging of the wrist. *Radiographics* 1989;9:229–246.

113. Quinn SF, Belsole RJ, Greene TL, Rayhack JM. Work in progress: Postarthrography computed tomography of the wrist—Evaluation of the triangular fibrocartilage complex. *Skeletal Radiol* 1989;17:565–569.

114. Quinn SF, Murray W, Watkins T, Kloss J. CT for determining the results of treatment of fractures of the wrist. *AJR* 1987;149:109–111.

115. Reicher MA, Kellerhouse LE. *MRI of the Wrist and Hand.* New York: Raven Press, 1990.

116. Reinus WR, Conway WF, Totty WG, et al. Carpal avascular necrosis: MR imaging. *Radiology* 1986;160:689–693.

117. Resnick D, Andre M, Kerr R, Pineda C, Guerra J Jr, Atkinson D. Digital arthrography of the wrist: A radiographic-pathologic investigation. *AJR* 1984;142:1187–1190.

118. Rettig AC. Stress fracture of the ulna in an adolescent tournament tennis player. *Am J Sports Med* 1983;11:103–106.

119. Rettig AC, Beltz HF. Stress fracture in the humerus in an adolescent tennis tournament player. *Am J Sports Med* 1985;13:55–58.

120. Rosen PR, Micheli LJ, Treves S. Early scintographic diagnosis of bone stress and fractures in athletic adolescents. *Pediatrics* 1982;70:11–15.

121. Roub LW, Gumerman LW, Hanley EN Jr, Clark MW, Goodman M, Herbert DL. Bone stress: A radionuclide imaging perspective. *Radiology* 1979;132:431–438.

122. Russe O. Fracture of the carpal navicular. Diagnosis, nonoperative treatment, and operative treatment. *J Bone Joint Surg* 1960;42A:759–768.

123. Sarrafian SK, Melamed JL, Goshgarian GM. Study of wrist motion in flexion and extension. *Clin Orthop* 1977;126:153–159.

124. Sclafani SJ. Dislocation of the distal radioulnar joint. *J Comput Assist Tomogr* 1981;5:450.

125. Skahen JR III, Palmer AK, Levinsohn EM, Buckingham SC, Szeverenyi NM. Magnetic resonance imaging of the triangular fibrocartilage complex. *J Hand Surg* 1990;15A:552–557.

126. Smith DK, Linscheid RL, Amadio PC, Berquist TH, Cooney WP. Scaphoid anatomy: Evaluation with complex motion tomography. *Radiology* 1989;173:177–180.

127. Smith FW, Gilday DL. Scintigraphic appearances of osteoid osteoma. *Radiology* 1980;137:191–195.

128. Solbiati L, Arsizio B, De Pra L, Rizzatto G, Derchi LE. High-resolution sonography in carpal tunnel syndrome. *Radiology* 1986;161(P):284.

129. Sowa DT, Holder LE, Patt PG, Weiland AJ. Application of magnetic resonance imaging to ischemic necrosis of the lunate. *J Hand Surg* 1989;14A:1008–1016.

130. Stahl F. Lunatomalacia (Kienböck's disease). A clinical and roentgenological study, especially on its pathogenesis and the late results of immobilization treatment. *Acta Chir Scand* 1947;95:1–133.

131. Stark HH, Jobe FW, Boyes JH, Ashworth CR. Fracture of the hook of the hamate in athletes. *J Bone Joint Surg* 1977;59A:575–582.

132. Stecher WR. Roentgenography of the carpal navicular bone. *AJR* 1937;37:704–705.
133. Subin GD, Mallon WJ, Urbaniak JR. Diagnosis of ganglion in Guyon's canal by magnetic resonance imaging. *J Hand Surg* 1989;14A:640–643.
134. Sy WM, Bay R, Camera A. Hand images: Normal and abnormal. *J Nucl Med* 1977;18:419–424.
135. Taleisnik J. Post-traumatic carpal instability. *Clin Orthop* 1980;419:73–82.
136. Tanz SS. Rotation effect in lunar and perilunar dislocations. *Clin Orthop* 1968;57:147–152.
137. Tehranzadeh J, Gabriele OF. Intra-articular calcified bodies: Detection by computed arthrotomography. *South Med J* 1984;77:703–710.
138. Terry DW Jr, Ramin JE. The navicular fat stripe: A useful roentgen feature for evaluating wrist trauma. *AJR* 1975;124:25–28.
139. Thomas HO. Isolated dislocation of the carpal scaphoid. *Acta Orthop Scand* 1977;48:369–372.
140. Tirman RM, Weber ER, Snyder LL, Koonce TW. Midcarpal wrist arthrography for detection of tears of the scapholunate and lunotriquetral ligaments. *AJR* 1985;144:107–108.
141. Totterman SM, Heberger R, Miller R, Rubens DJ, Blebea JS. Two-piece wrist surface coil. *AJR* 1991;156:343–344.
142. Trentham DE, Hamm RL, Masi AT. Wrist arthrography: Review and comparison of normals, rheumatoid arthritis and gout patients. *Semin Arthritis Rheum* 1975;5:105–120.
143. Trumble TE. Avascular necrosis after scaphoid fracture: A correlation of magnetic resonance imaging and histology. *J Hand Surg* 1990;15A:557–564.
144. Verdan C. Fractures of the scaphoid. *Surg Clin North Am* 1960;40:461–464.
145. Viegas SF, Ballantyne G. Attritional lesions of the wrist joint. *J Hand Surg* 1987;12A:1025–1029.
146. Voorhees DR, Daffner RH, Nunley JA, Gilula LA. Carpal ligamentous disruptions and negative ulnar variance. *Skeletal Radiol* 1985;13:257–262.
147. Wagner CJ. Fracture-dislocations of the wrist. *Clin Orthop* 1959;15:181–196.
148. Wahner HW. Radionuclides in the diagnosis of fracture healing. *J Nucl Med* 1978;19:1356–1358.
149. Wechsler RJ, Wehbe MA, Rifkin MD, Edeiken J, Branch HM. Computed tomography diagnosis of distal radioulnar subluxation. *Skeletal Radiol* 1987;16:1–5.
150. Weiss KL, Beltran J, Shamam OM, Stilla RF, Levey M. High-field MR surface-coil imaging of the hand and wrist. I. Normal anatomy. *Radiology* 1986;160:143–146.
151. Weiss C, Laskin RS, Spinner M. Irreducible trans-scaphoid perilunate dislocation. *J Bone Joint Surg* 1970;52A:565–568.
152. Weseley MS, Barenfeld PA. Trans-scaphoid, transcapitate, transtriquetral, perilunate fracture–dislocation of the wrist. A case report. *J Bone Joint Surg* 1972;54A:1073–1078.
153. White SJ, Louis DS, Braunstein EM, Hankin FM, Greene TL. Capitate-lunate instability: Recognition by manipulation under fluoroscopy. *AJR* 1984;143:361–364.
154. Wilson AJ, Gilula LA, Mann FA. Unidirectional joint communications in wrist arthrography: An evaluation of 250 cases. *AJR* 1991;157:105–109.
155. Wilson JN. Profiles of the carpal canal. *J Bone Joint Surg* 1954;36A:127–132.
156. Woodward AH, Neviaser RJ, Nisenfeld F. Radial and volar perilunate transscaphoid fracture dislocation. *South Med J* 1975;68:926–928.
157. Yeager BA, Dalinka MK. Radiology of trauma to the wrist: dislocations, fracture dislocations, and instability patterns. *Skeletal Radiol* 1985;13:120–130.
158. Zeiss J, Skie M, Ebraheim N, Jackson WT. Anatomic relations between the median nerve and flexor tendons in the carpal tunnel: MR evaluation in normal volunteers. *AJR* 1989;153:533–536.
159. Zlatkin MB, Chao PC, Osterman AL, Schnall MD, Dalinka MK, Kressel HY. Chronic wrist pain: evaluation with high-resolution MR imaging. *Radiology* 1989;173:723–729.
160. Zucker-Pinchoff B, Hermann G, Srinivasan R. Computed tomography of the carpal tunnel: A radioanatomic study. *J Comput Assist Tomogr* 1981;5:525–528.

Wrist Arthroscopy Equipment, Operating Room Set-Up, and the Surgical Team

Judy L. Cooper, M.D., *Gary G. Poehling*, M.D., *Stephen J. Chabon*, P.A.-C., *and L. Andrew Koman*, M.D.

Arthroscopy of the wrist is equipment- and environment-dependent. Specialized tools and a knowledgeable surgical team are required to accomplish this complex and demanding diagnostic and therapeutic procedure (1–10). This chapter describes the role of the surgical team and the currently available equipment, preparation, and positioning of the patient. Cameras and light sources are not included because they are standard equipment for all arthroscopic procedures.

ROOM ARRANGEMENT

The operating room should be arranged to accommodate all necessary equipment for the procedure. The surgical bed is positioned with the anesthetist at the head of the table. An arm board or narrow hand table is placed on the operative side of the surgical table, and sitting stools are positioned on each side of the arm board. The electronic video center is opposite the operative side for ease in viewing the procedure. The instrument table is positioned at the end of the arm board for easy access. Other accessory equipment is located on the opposite side of the surgical table to decrease clutter around the sterile surgical field.

When preparing the sterile table, an arthroscopy pack is used. This is effective in exposing the wrist joint for any procedure undertaken. After the skin prep is completed, an impervious sheet is placed on the arm board or hand table for extra protection and fluid containment. A stockinette is placed over the hand and rolled above the elbow, and the extremity sheet is positioned. The stockinette is then cut at the top and folded down to the opening of the extremity sheet, exposing the hand and wrist. Coban is used to create a tight seal around the stockinette and sheet and to resist fluid extravasation into the forearm. The arm is now ready for application of the sterile finger traps and attachment of the traction method preferred. If a sterile traction tower is used, its base is placed beneath the patient's elbow with the upright parallel to the forearm (Fig. 1).

Instruments on the sterile table should be positioned in order of use. Instrument cords that need to be connected to the video source and passed to the nonsterile field should be free of knots, and all electrical connections must be dried thoroughly.

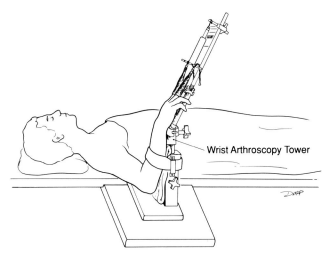

FIG. 1. The wrist tower with disposable finger traps, a spring-loaded traction device with tension gauge, and a ball joint, which allows specialized position changes.

SURGICAL TEAM

The surgical team should be coordinated from the preparation of the surgical suite through the transporting of the patient to the recovery room. When all members are familiar with the procedures and the equipment needed, the smooth functioning and efficiency of the procedure are greatly enhanced. Assigning specific responsibilities to each member on the team ensures that all tasks are completed. Repetition and consistency of the procedure also add to increased efficiency and coordination of the team.

Circulator

The circulator prepares, coordinates, and maintains all necessary supportive functions throughout the procedure. Ideally, there should be two circulators in the surgical suite for the rapid completion of the many necessary tasks.

After the sterile field is established, irrigation tubing is connected to lactated Ringer's solution, and suction tubing, light cable, camera cord, and power shaver connections are passed to the circulator to be hooked up to their sources. Fine adjustments at each source are accomplished in cooperation with the scrub nurse.

Video recording and still photography are the responsibility of the circulating nurse. All necessary attachments required to obtain the image should be connected to the camera. Sterile attachments to be used should be given to the scrub nurse for adequate preparation.

During the procedure, the circulator must be attentive to any need that may arise. Monitoring the progress of the procedure and anticipating needs can greatly enhance optimal team functioning and efficiency.

A record of all pertinent events is kept by the circulator during the surgical procedure: patient positioning; tourniquet time; specimens; instrument, needle, and sponge counts in the event of an open procedure; operating times; anesthesia needs; and equipment charges. This record is the legal document that describes the patient's care while in the surgical suite, and the record must be both accurate and complete.

Scrub Nurse

The primary duty of the scrub nurse is to maintain the sterile environment. The scrub nurse should be knowledgeable of the procedure being performed. This includes the equipment and instruments that are indicated for use and any special conditions the surgeon may have requested to facilitate the smooth functioning of the procedure. Directing the circulator to any needs that must be met and anticipating the needs of the surgeon will facilitate the procedure and eliminate unnecessary frustrations.

The instruments must be cleaned each time they are withdrawn from the joint. This will remove any tissue debris and prevent unwanted fragments from reentering the joint. The importance of regular instrument inspection for breakage, wear, corrosion, or fatigue cannot be overemphasized, for it can prevent a very unnecessary delay factor of arthroscopic surgery. Specimens must be handled carefully, and passed to the circulator for proper preparation and labeling for the laboratory.

Assistant

The primary responsibility of the assistant is to facilitate the effectiveness and efficiency of the surgeon. This position can be filled by the scrub nurse or another trained assistant.

The assistant must understand the procedure and the objective to be achieved. Understanding of the arthroscopic anatomy and pathology of the wrist greatly enhances the ability of the assistant to anticipate the surgeon's actions and to share information with other members of the surgical team.

Mental and manual synchrony with the surgeon is the optimal goal of the assistant at all times during the procedure. Any actions of the surgeon that the assistant is unfamiliar with should be addressed immediately so that optimal coordination can be maintained.

Assisting with the position of the wrist in flexion, extension, and radial and ulnar deviation or applying gentle counterpressure on the wrist aids the surgeon in establishing entry portals and inserting the appropriate instruments.

There are times when the surgeon may need to visualize the anatomy, as well as to use both hands to perform the surgical procedure. The assistant may need to steady the arthroscope for the surgeon and maintain the needed image within the center of the visual field.

Other functions of the assistant include avoiding excessive weight on the tubing and electrical cords, removing unnecessary instruments, and avoiding cord tangles.

Supporting instruments, inserting wires, and holding cannulas and retractors when necessary are possible duties of the assistant. If an open surgical procedure is indicated, the assistant must maintain visual and manual access for the surgeon's operative maneuvers. In effect, the assistant is the surgeon's second pair of hands, and he or she should coordinate with the surgeon's intentions as naturally and spontaneously as possible.

The operating room is a complex environment. Wrist arthroscopy with its innovative and evolving surgical techniques dictates new challenges for the surgical team. Team coordination and consistency are essential to optimal efficiency in performing any surgical procedure. Attention to detail, knowledge of the procedure, and established responsibilities of each team member are vital to achieving successful goals in wrist arthroscopy.

ARTHROSCOPES

The most critical piece of equipment in wrist arthroscopy is, of course, the arthroscope (Fig. 2). Its diameter should range from 1.6 to 3.0 mm. The smaller diameter arthroscopes fit easily within the joint spaces but are more fragile and have a smaller and dimmer field of view, dimmer because they contain fewer fiberoptic light bundles. Larger diameter arthroscopes have an increased field of view and a brighter image, but their mobility is significantly restricted, particularly in the midcarpal and distal radial ulnar joints.

The length of the arthroscope should be appropriate to the size of the structure under view. To accommodate all sizes of wrists, the arthroscope should be 40–60 mm long. If it is shorter than 40 mm, the depths of larger wrists may not be visualized. The longer arthroscopes have the disadvantage of fragility, which increases as the length increases and the diameter decreases.

A critical feature of the arthroscope is its angle of vision. The curvature of the bones and articular surfaces of

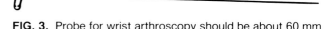

FIG. 3. Probe for wrist arthroscopy should be about 60 mm in length and 1.5 mm in diameter.

the wrist cannot be evaluated properly unless the arthroscope has an angle of vision of at least 25°. Another variable is how the image is presented to the camera or to the eye. If the arthroscope has an eyepiece, the joint may be seen directly through the telescope. However, a camera adaptor must be added if television equipment is to be used. Alternatively, a camera adaptor is unnecessary for the arthroscope without an eyepiece. The absence of an eyepiece is an advantage, because the fewer the interfaces presented to the camera, the brighter and clearer the picture is on the television screen. The disadvantages are that without an eyepiece the surgeon cannot look directly through the telescope, and a 35-mm photograph cannot be taken directly through it.

HAND INSTRUMENTS

Needles

A needle is used to localize the joint at the beginning of the procedure. A needle causes minimal tissue trauma and is very effective in locating the position of portal sites and ensuring that the placement of a portal allows appropriate access to the injured area.

I generally use an 18-gauge, $1\frac{1}{2}$-inch needle attached to a 20-cc syringe filled with lactated Ringer's solution. Subsequent joint distention ensures proper placement for the initial approach to the wrist. Distension of the joint separates the articular surfaces and minimizes articular scuffing during the initial insertion of the arthroscope. Once the arthroscope is in the joint, the insertion of an 18-gauge needle in the 6R portal may be observed directly. This may serve as a gravity inflow portal, or if a mechanical pump is being used, it may serve as a marker for insertion of the outflow and pressure-sensing cannula. An instrument portal should be established in the 4–5 site, through which a probe may be inserted to palpate the structures within the joint during the initial visualization.

Probes

The probe is the most frequently used instrument in wrist arthroscopy (Fig. 3). It should be blunt and rounded to prevent damage to the articular cartilage and should measure 1–2 mm in diameter and 40–60 mm in length. The probe is especially useful during the diagnostic portion of wrist arthroscopy. By providing a scale for size comparison, as well as providing tactile feedback,

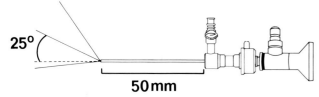

FIG. 2. Critical dimensions of a wrist arthroscope are less than 3 mm in diameter and 40–60 mm in length, and have a 25–30° angle of vision.

the probe aids in the accurate assessment of normal and abnormal anatomy of the joint. The feedback helps to distinguish the triangular fibrocartilage (rubbery feeling) from the distal radius (firm feeling) and in locating the intercarpal ligaments. Probably its most important role is to serve as a palpating finger in search of hidden disease, such as a triangular fibrocartilage tear or dynamic ligament instability.

Basket Forceps

Basket forceps for use in the wrist have been adapted from instruments used in the knee. The basket forceps (Fig. 4A) should be 2–3 mm in diameter and 40–60 mm long. The tip should be square, with the largest cutting surface at the front of the instrument. The lower jaw should be narrow and yet strong enough that the tissue to be cut can be placed in the open jaws with minimal displacement. This design provides maximal cutting efficiency and minimal space displacement, while maintaining strength and durability. A "cowcatcher" (Fig. 4B) may be useful in positioning the instrument for trimming a triangular fibrocartilage tear. A "scissors" grip is the most appropriate design for performing these delicate tasks.

Grasping Forceps

The grasping forceps (Fig. 4C) should be 2–3 mm in diameter. Because of the many curved surfaces in the wrist joint, a slight curve to the jaws is advantageous.

Ronguers

A rongeur (Fig. 4D) is particularly useful in removing joint debris and portions of carpal bones. It should be about 3 mm in diameter and have a smooth, rounded tip.

Curettes

Curettes are occasionally useful in trimming the edges of loose articular cartilage.

Knives

Some surgeons prefer to use knives to trim the triangular fibrocartilage. Hook knives and banana blades seem to be the most efficient designs for wrist arthroscopy.

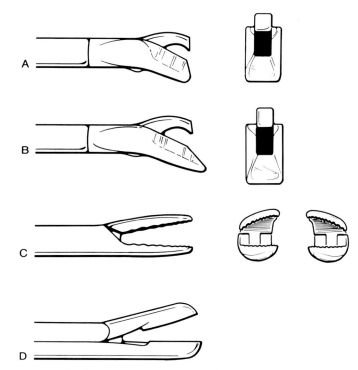

FIG. 4. Profile and head-on views of cutting and grasping tools. **A:** Basket forceps for the wrist should maximize cutting efficiency and minimize space displacement. **B:** Wrist basket forceps with lower jaw tongue ("cowcatcher"). **C:** Grasping forceps. **D:** Rongeur.

POWER INSTRUMENTS

Power equipment permits rapid morselization of tissue within the joint. Most power devices include a suction aspiration system for evacuation of tissue particles. This is a great advantage because small chips of tissue left within the joint space may provoke an inflammatory reaction or interfere mechanically with joint function postoperatively.

Size and Balance

Due to the unique configuration and limited space in the wrist, instruments may be inserted to a depth of only 10–15 mm. The pivotal fulcrum provided by the joint capsule is located relatively close to the tip of the instrument. Long instruments and heavy hand pieces produce a greater bending moment on the small diameter of the instrument shafts. This not only places an unnecessary strain on the instrument, with bending of the rotating shafts and possible introduction of metallic debris in the joint, but it is also very tiring for the arthroscopist.

Appropriate balance of the hand piece is important when time-consuming and tedious procedures are to be performed, and it should be a primary consideration when selecting power equipment.

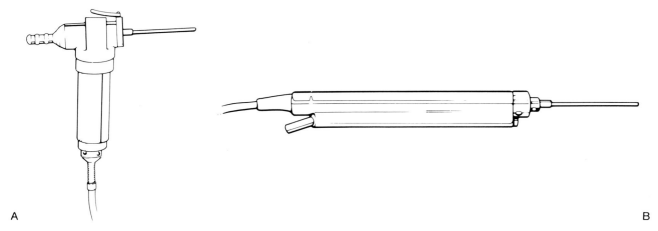

A   B

FIG. 5. Power instruments are designed with either a pistol (**A**) or a pencil (**B**) grip.

Grips

Power instruments have either a pistol (Fig. 5A) or a pencil (Fig. 5B) grip. The pistol grip is most appropriate for instruments that require strength from the ulnar side of the arthroscopist's hand. With this grip, the weight should be concentrated in the handle and the center of the palm. The pencil grip takes advantage of the superior fine motor movement of the thumb, index, and long fingers and enhances precision maneuvers.

Tips

The morselizing ability of a tip depends on the degree to which the tip is covered. Because the volume of the wrist is small, synovitis may obscure the arthroscopist's vision. A relatively covered tip (Fig. 6A) is then useful, because it eliminates the possibility of cutting any firm tissue. Only the more delicate synovial tissue is thus removed, providing improved visualization of the joint. However, when visualization is excellent and the tissue is firm, such as when an articular cartilage flap or the end of a torn ligament is to be cut, an uncovered tip (Fig. 6B) is more efficient.

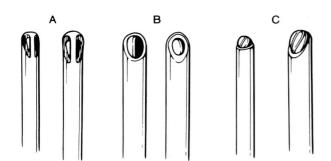

A   B   C

FIG. 6. Tips used in power instruments: covered (**A**), uncovered (**B**), and round (**C**) burs.

Burs

Miniature power burs (Fig. 6C) are effective in the management of osseous lesions, such as eburnated articular surfaces or osteophytes.

Mechanical Pumps

One of the major problems encountered in arthroscopy of small joints is balancing fluid inflow and outflow. With only 5–7 ml of total volume, a snug arthroscope sheath, and an inflow cannula using an 18- or 20-gauge needle, the dependency of a gravity flow system on the suction control provided by power instruments causes problems during surgery and is unsatisfactory in many cases. Alternatively, a mechanical pump can be used to allow inflow through the sheath of the arthroscope in sufficient volume to balance the inflow and outflow during the use of instruments that depend on suction (Fig. 7). Ideally, this could be accomplished using two portals and still allow instrument utilization in the second portal. A third monitoring portal is not difficult to use in the radiocarpal joint, but it is difficult in the midcarpal joint. We believe that we will see greater utilization of mechanical pumps in the future, especially in small-joint arthroscopy, in which the ability to balance inflow and outflow while maintaining a relatively constant pressure is most needed.

Controls

The initiation and direction of rotation of the tip of the arthroscope is generally controlled from the hand piece or by a foot pedal. Having an oscillating mode that reverses the direction of the cutting blade at short intervals is advantageous, because this seems to increase the efficiency of cutting. Control of suction on instru-

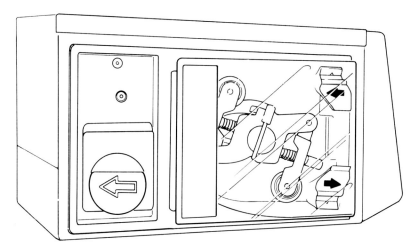

FIG. 7. Mechanical pump designed to balance inflow and outflow and maintain a relatively constant pressure.

ments is important when regulation of the amount of fluid inflow is limited. The critical factor is to balance inflow and outflow. If a mechanical pump is used, inflow can be increased to match outflow, and control of suction is less critical. If a gravity flow system is used, however, the suction control on the hand piece maintains fluid balance.

ACCESSORIES

Finger Traps

Finger traps are standard equipment for wrist arthroscopy procedures. Sterilized finger traps are positioned over the PIP joint on the prepped fingers (generally the index and long fingers) and attached to a positioning device. If the problem is primarily on the ulnar side, the traps may be placed on the little and ring fingers. Care must be taken in placing the traps on fingers that have weakened or delicate skin.

Suspension Devices

Overhead Boom

The overhead boom is a series of pulleys, which are usually attached to the operating table to provide traction on the extremity (Fig. 8).

Stabilization

The wrist may be stabilized by using a forearm bar that is connected to the operating table, or by adding countertraction over a felt loop on the upper arm (Fig. 8). The

forearm bar secures and supports the arm as it is being prepped. If an open operation is necessary, however, the arm must be reprepped and redraped. Although the felt loop countertraction technique provides less security, it provides more flexibility during the operative procedure.

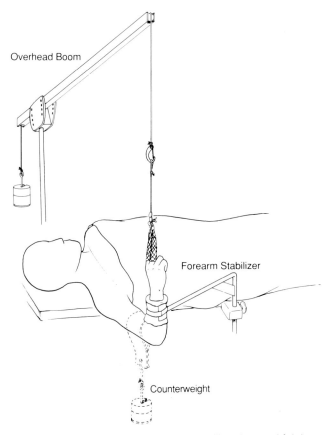

FIG. 8. Overhead boom with wrist stabilizer bar and felt loop countertraction (*broken lines*).

Arthrobot

The arthrobot was developed from robotic technology. It is controlled by electricity, powered by compressed air, and has a variety of grasping devices. For the wrist, finger traps are used. The arthrobot is covered by a sterile plastic bag, which allows easy changes in wrist position during surgery. The release controls are activated by grasping the instrument in the control area and placing the instrument and the patient's hand in the desired position. Releasing the control area freezes the instrument in place, securing the position of the extremity. The primary advantage of the arthrobot is its versatility.

Wrist Traction Tower

The traction tower is the newest innovation for applying traction to the wrist joint during wrist arthroscopy (see Fig. 1). It has the advantage of being completely sterile, and it provides great flexibility of wrist position. It is the only device that allows continued traction with the wrist joint in flexion, a position that opens the dorsal aspect of the wrist and allows easier insertion of the equipment into the radiocarpal and midcarpal joints.

REFERENCES

1. Botte MJ, Cooney WP, Linscheid RL. Arthroscopy of the wrist: Anatomy and technique. *J Hand Surg* 1989;14:313–316.
2. Dutka M. Elbow and wrist arthroscopy: Perioperative nursing care. *Orthop Nurs* 1986;5:29–34.
3. Nichols CD. Wrist arthroscopy. An ambulatory surgery procedure. *AORN J* 1989;49:759–763,766,768.
4. Poehling GG. Wrist arthroscopy. Portals to progress. In: *An Illustrated Guide to Small Joint Arthroscopy.* Andover, MA: Dyonics, Inc., pp. 7–12.
5. Poehling GG, Roth J, Whipple T, Koman LA, Toby B. *Arthroscopic Surgery of the Wrist. Information Manual.* Winston-Salem, NC: Bowman Gray School of Medicine.
6. Roth JH. Radiocarpal arthroscopy. *Orthopedics* 1988;11:1309–1312.
7. Roth JH, Poehling GG, Whipple TL. Arthroscopic surgery of the wrist. *Instr Course Lect* 1988;37:183–194.
8. Toby EB, Poehling GG, Koman AL. Midcarpal arthroscopy. *Surg Rounds Orthop* 1989;3:23–27.
9. Whipple TL. Power instruments for wrist arthroscopy. *Arthroscopy* 1988;4:290–294.
10. Whipple TL, Marotta JJ, Powell JH III. Techniques of wrist arthroscopy. *Arthroscopy* 1986;2:244–252.

Surgical Technique for Wrist Arthroscopy

Terry L. Whipple, M.D., *Gary G. Poehling*, M.D., *and James H. Roth*, M.D.

For both diagnostic and therapeutic arthroscopy, the patient is placed in a supine position. General, intravenous regional, or brachial block anesthesia is administered. The patient's shoulder is then abducted 90° with the arm resting on two parallel arm boards or a hand table.

After antiseptic skin preparation and sterile draping, finger traps are applied. Finger traps are placed on the index and long fingers for general diagnostic examinations and also when disease or trauma is suspected on the radial side of the wrist. When a specific lesion is suspected on the ulnar side of the wrist, finger traps may be applied to the ulnar digits. The finger traps should cover the proximal intraphalangeal joints to avoid slippage. The patient's elbow is flexed 90° with the forearm vertical, and traction is applied (6 to 10 pounds, depending on the patient's size). Use of the traction tower (Fig. 1) is preferred for simplicity and stability.

Unless disease or trauma on the ulnar side of the wrist has been confirmed preoperatively, the arthroscope is inserted in the 3–4 portal. The 4–5, 1–2, 6U, and 6R portals are available for the introduction of accessory instruments and an inflow cannula (Fig. 2). If ulnar disease is suspected or confirmed preoperatively, the arthroscope is introduced into the 6R portal, and accessory instruments and the inflow cannula are used in the 3–4, 1–2, 4–5, or 6U portal.

Irrigation requires a physiologic solution. Lactated Ringer's solution appears most compatible with hyaline cartilage, although normal saline solution may also be used. The procedure is begun by injecting 5–7 ml of irrigating solution into the radiocarpal space through the 3–4 portal. The inflow cannula is then placed in an appropriate portal. Backflow of irrigating fluid confirms entry of the catheter into the radiocarpal space. Care should be taken to flush all air bubbles from the tubing before it is connected to the inflow cannula. The skin is then lanced over the 3–4 portal. A blunt trocar and a cannula are inclined proximally to parallel the volar tilt of the articular surface of the radius. With pressure and a twisting motion, the trocar and cannula are inserted into the radiocarpal space.

The camera and telescope assembly are inserted into the joint through the cannula. Distention of the joint is maintained by irrigating fluid through the inflow cannula with outflow through the arthroscope sheath (1–8). Alternatively, a mechanical fluid pump can be connected to the sheath of the arthroscope with a pressure monitor and outflow line connected to the cannula (Fig. 3).

An initial, cursory examination of the radiocarpal space should include visualization of the articular surface of the radius and the triangular fibrocartilage articular disc (TFC), the articular surface of the proximal carpal row, and the volar capsule and ligaments. Selection of an accessory portal is based on the location of any apparent abnormality noticed during this preliminary examination. A probe is usually inserted in the 4–5 portal, but the 1–2 or the 6R portal may be appropriate. The best accessory portal can be identified by placing a 21-gauge needle through the skin under arthroscopic visualization to ensure that the pathologic area can be reached by the intended portal.

Keeping the tip of the probe in sight and palpating all surfaces to appreciate texture, tension, and any disruption of otherwise smooth surfaces, the arthroscopist repeats the examination of the joint in deliberate fashion. The wrist may be flexed, extended, or deviated to the radial or ulnar side to improve visualization, if necessary.

Directly in front of the 3–4 portal on the volar side of the joint is a tuft of synovium, arising consistently at the volar end of the scapholunate ligament, which acts as a landmark (Fig. 4). To the radial side of this tuft are the radiolunotriquetral ligament and the radioscaphocapitate ligament (Fig. 5). To the ulnar side are the ulnolunate and ulnotriquetral ligaments. If the synovial tuft is retracted to one side, sometimes the short radioscapholunate ligament of Testut can be visualized.

The articular surfaces of the proximal pole of scaphoid and of the lunate are convex. Between them, in the normal state, a slight reversal of this convex contour indicates the location of the scapholunate ligament (Fig. 6). Further to the ulnar side, the proximal pole of the

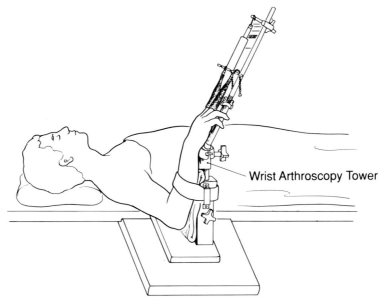

FIG. 1. Traction tower allows for distraction and wrist flexion, which simplifies the arthroscopic procedure.

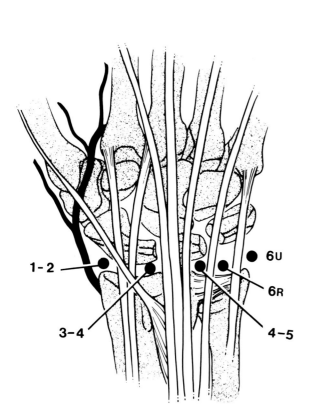

FIG. 2. Routine portals of the radiocarpal joint.

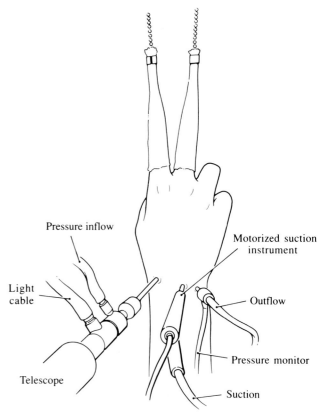

FIG. 3. Effective operative instrumentation of the radiocarpal joint needs to include pressurized inflow through the telescope as well as accommodating outflow and pressure monitoring. This allows the effective use of suction instruments within this very small joint.

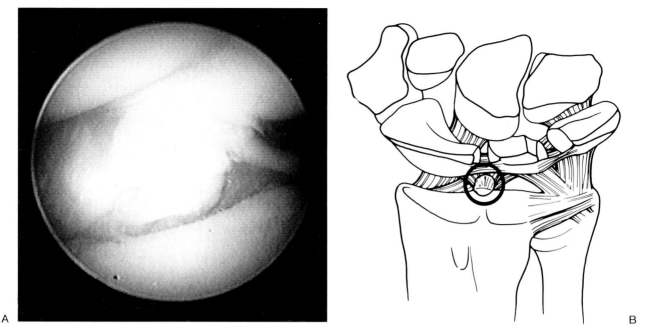

FIG. 4. A, B: Fat pad over the radioscapholunate ligament just under the volar aspect of the scapholunate ligament.

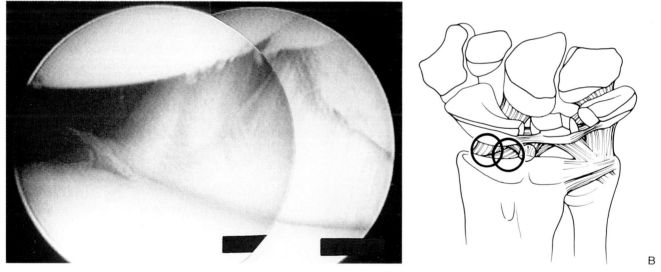

FIG. 5. A, B: The radioscaphocapitate ligament is most radial, with the radiolunotriquetral just to its ulnar side.

triquetrum can be visualized along with a glimpse of the lunotriquetral ligament.

Proximally, the scaphoid facet of the radius is separated from the lunate facet by the sagittal ridge (Fig. 7). It is not unusual for this ridge to exhibit slight fraying of the hyaline cartilage. Attached firmly to the lunate facet articular cartilage is the TFC. In the normal wrist, the transition from lunate facet to TFC can best be appreciated by palpation with a probe (Fig. 8).

After complete examination through the 3–4 portal, the arthroscope should be moved to the 6R portal with a probe transferred to the 3–4 portal. This will allow thorough visualization of the ulnar side of the joint, with better inspection of the lunotriquetral ligament, the articular surface of the triquetrum, and the volar ulnocarpal ligaments (Fig. 9). The opening in the ulnar joint capsule represents the entry into the prestyloid recess. Sometimes, either through this opening or through a secondary opening slightly more volar, the arthroscopist can see the ulnar margin of the articulation between the pisiform and the triquetrum (Fig. 10).

Arthroscopic examination of the midcarpal space

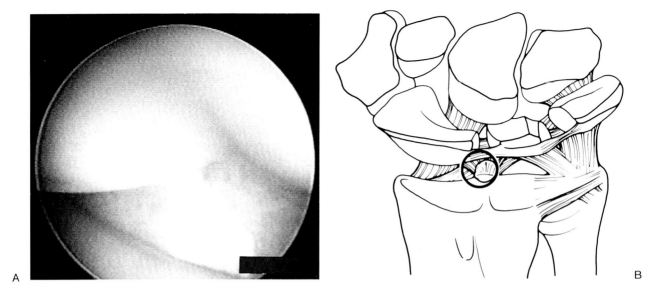

FIG. 6. A, B: In many patients the scapholunate ligament is concave.

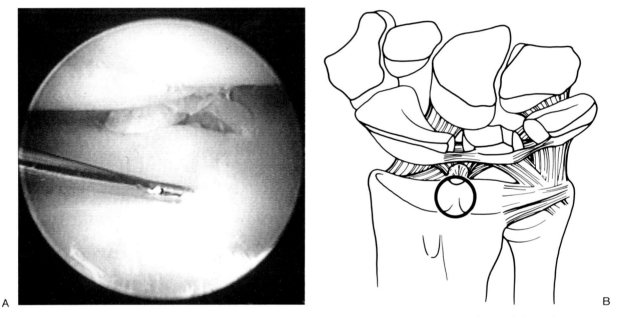

FIG. 7. A, B: Sagittal ridge is the division between the scaphoid facet and the lunate facet of the radius.

should be routine. The sheath of the arthroscope and the trocar are introduced through the radial midcarpal portal after the overlying skin is lanced (Fig. 11). The inflow tubing should be connected to the sheath of the arthroscope for the introduction of the irrigating solution. When the arthroscope is inserted into the sheath, the concave surface of the scaphoid can be seen opposite the convex head of the capitate (Fig. 12). A systematic examination of the midcarpal space should include evaluation of the articular surfaces of the scaphotrapeziotrapezoid (STT) joint (Fig. 13) distally and to the radial midcarpal side of the portal. If necessary, an accessory instrument

can be introduced through the STT portal to facilitate this examination. To the ulnar side, the examination should include the articular margins of the scapholunate interval (Fig. 14), the alignment of the scaphoid and lunate, the articulations and alignment of the lunotriquetral joint (Fig. 15), the articular surfaces of the capitate, and the proximal pole of the hamate (Fig. 16). The laxity of the saddle-shaped triquetrohamate joint should be tested, and the attachment of the dorsal capsule to the hamate and capitate should be inspected.

The ulnar midcarpal portal can be used for introduction of accessory instruments on the ulnar side of the

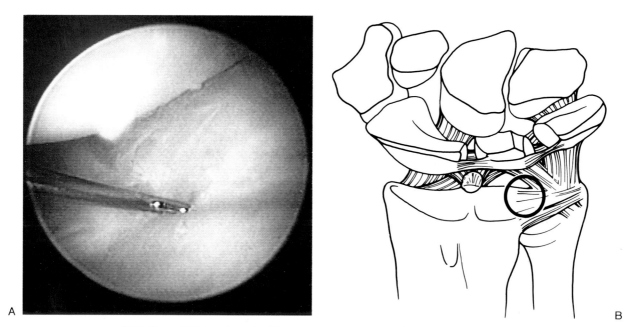

FIG. 8. A, B: The triangular fibrocartilage is best appreciated by palpation.

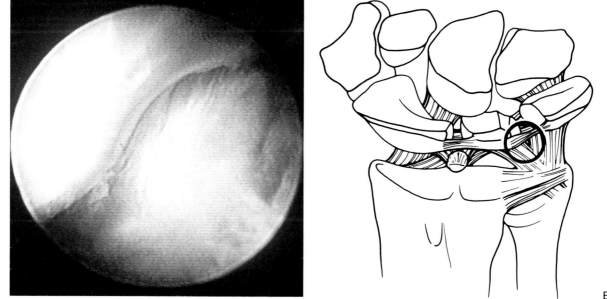

FIG. 9. A, B: The ulnotriquetral and ulnolunate ligaments are best seen from the ulnar portals.

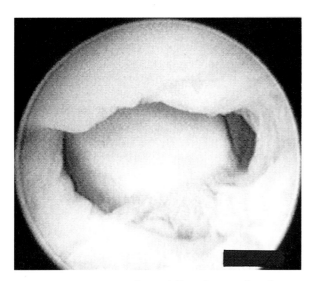

FIG. 10. Visualization of the pisiform is occasionally possible in the normal wrist. If it is very evident, one must consider an ulnotriquetral ligament tear as the reason for its visibility.

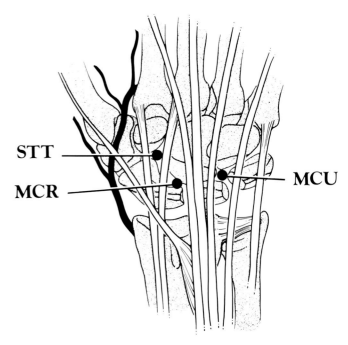

FIG. 11. There are three midcarpal portals, scaphotrapezio-trapezoid (STT), midcarpal radial (MCR), and midcarpal ulnar (MCU).

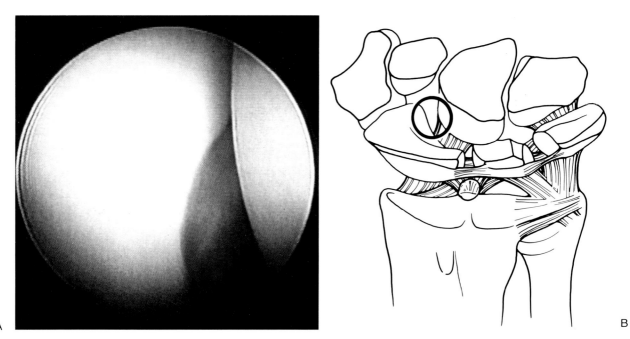

A

B

FIG. 12. A, B: The scaphoid is to the left and the capitate is to the right.

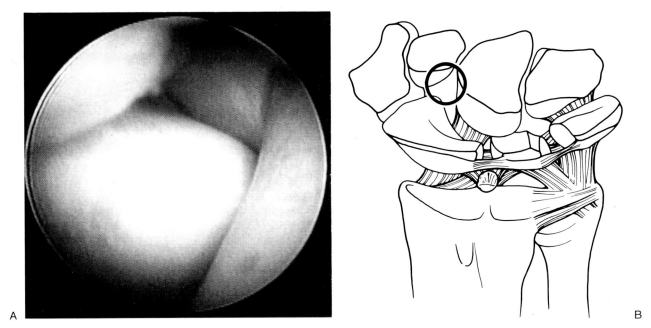

FIG. 13. A, B: Scaphotrapeziotrapezoid (STT) joint seen through the midcarpal radial (MCR) portal.

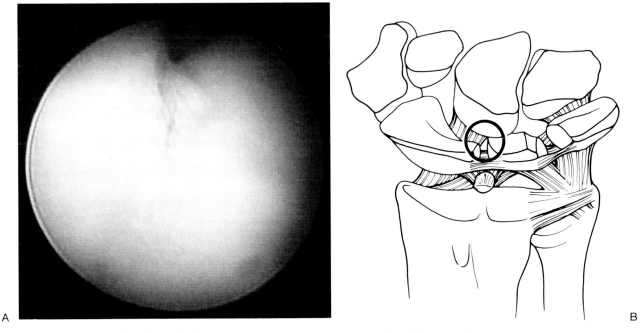

FIG. 14. A, B: The scapholunate joint seen through the midcarpal radial portal.

midcarpal space. Conversely, the arthroscope can be transferred to the ulnar midcarpal portal with accessory instruments being used in the radial midcarpal portal.

Finally, the distal radioulnar joint is examined in selected cases. This is a difficult joint to enter in the small wrist, but the attempt should be made when the clinical symptoms warrant an examination. The dorsal wrist should be held in supination, which relaxes the dorsal

capsule of the distal radioulnar joint (DRUJ). After identifying the DRUJ-1 or DRUJ-2 portal (Fig. 17), the joint can be distended by injecting about 1.5 ml of irrigating solution with a hypodermic needle. The skin is then lanced and the arthroscope sheath with blunt trocar is twisted gently but firmly into the DRUJ. Through the DRUJ-1 portal, the sheath enters between the head of the ulna and the TFC. This portal should only be utilized

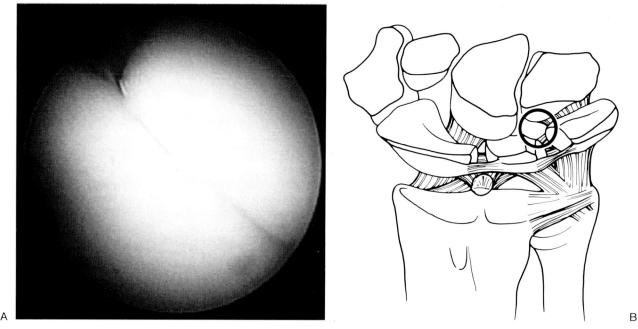

FIG. 15. A, B: The lunotriquetral joint seen through the MCR portal.

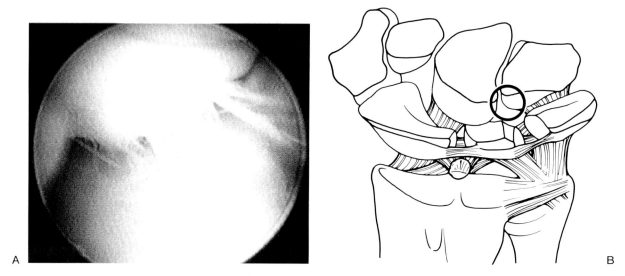

FIG. 16. A, B: Chondromalacia of the tip of the hamate.

for patients in whom radiographs demonstrate at least some degree of negative ulnar variance. The DRUJ-2 portal enters in the axilla of the radius and ulna. When the arthroscope is introduced into the portal through the sheath, the metaphyseal portion of the ulna can be seen readily, and the sigmoid notch of the radius can be identified distally. Gentle pronation and supination of the wrist will move the articular margin of the head of the ulna in front of the arthroscope to expose any degenerative articular changes present.

Before withdrawing the arthroscope from any of the above three joint spaces, the arthroscopist may elect to inject 1–2 ml of bupivacaine to reduce postoperative discomfort.

A sterile compressive bandage is applied to cover the portals. A splint may be used for comfort for 1–5 days.

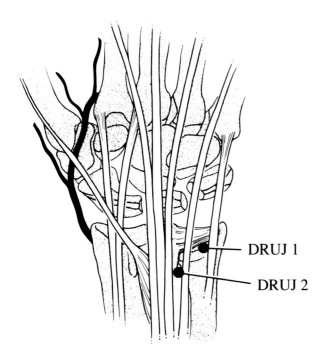

FIG. 17. Portals to the distal radioulnar joint (DRUJ).

DRUJ 1

DRUJ 2

REFERENCES

1. Cooney WP. Arthroscopy of the wrist. Anatomy and classification of carpal instability. *Arthroscopy* 1990;2:133–140.
2. Osterman AL. Arthroscopic debridement of the triangular fibrocartilage tears. *Arthroscopy* 1990;2:120–124.
3. Palmer AK. Triangular fibrocartilage afflications: injury patterns and treatment. *Arthroscopy* 1990;2:125–132.
4. Poehling GG. Wrist arthroscopy: portals to progress. In: *An Illustrated Guide to Small Joint Arthroscopy.* Andover, MA: Dyonics, Inc., 1989;7–12.
5. Poehling GG, Roth J, Whipple T, Koman LA, Toby B. *Arthroscopic Surgery of the Wrist. Information Manual.* Winston-Salem, NC: Bowman Gray School of Medicine.
6. Roth JH, Haddad RG. Radiocarpal arthroscopy and arthrography in the diagnosis of ulnar wrist pain. *Arthroscopy* 1986;2:234–243.
7. Roth JH, Poehling GG, Whipple TL. Arthroscopic surgery of the wrist. *Inst Course Lect* 1988;37:183–194.
8. Whipple TL, Marotta JJ, Powell JH III. Techniques of wrist arthroscopy. *Arthroscopy* 1986;2:244–252.

Carpal Instabilities

Gary G. Poehling, M.D., *Stephen J. Chabon*, P.A.-C., *and David S. Ruch*, M.D.

In their 1972 landmark article, Linscheid, Dobyns, and coauthors defined traumatic instability of the wrist as "a carpal injury in which loss of normal alignment of the carpal bones developed early or late." Four major malalignments were recognized: dorsiflexion, palmar flexion, ulnar translocation, and dorsal subluxation (3). Since that time, our understanding of the causes of carpal instabilities has continued to advance. The arthroscope has further enhanced that understanding and, in certain instances, has allowed minimally invasive techniques to correct the encountered lesion.

CLASSIFICATION

At the 1987 meeting of the American Academy of Orthopaedic Surgeons in San Francisco, Dobyns reported a division of carpal instabilities into two groups, which are in standard usage today. The first and most common group was termed a carpal instability, dissociative (CID), and these instabilities are seen with tears of the scapholunate ligament and the lunotriquetral ligament (2). It is for this group of injuries that arthroscopy has the greatest impact, and they will be the major focus of this chapter. The second group was termed carpal instability, nondissociative (CIND), a much less common group of instabilities. The CIND lesion involves the ulnoarcuate ligament complex on the palmar side of the wrist, with the instability existing between the proximal and the distal

carpal rows. This type of instability has been termed a capitolunate instability pattern (CLIP) or, as described in Chapter 7 (*this volume*), a palmar midcarpal instability (PMCI) (2).

HISTORY OF CARPAL INSTABILITY, DISSOCIATIVE (CID)

Classically, injuries to the scapholunate and lunotriquetral ligaments are the result of trauma. Mayfield, Johnson, and Kilcoyne, in 1980, stated that intercarpal supination was the major factor in the initial production of a scapholunate dissociation (4). Five years later, Talesnik stated that it was carpal hyperpronation with loading of the ulnar side of the carpus that resulted in lunotriquetral injury (5). Over the last 4–5 years, with the help of the arthroscope, we have been able to define a spectrum of these carpal ligament injuries. The trauma causing these injuries has ranged from a very mild twisting injury to a severe impact from falls or a direct blow sustained in a motor vehicle accident. Frequently, the preliminary roentgenograms have been normal or the lesion has not been recognized, and it is only when symptoms persist that the patient is seen by the wrist surgeon. Usually, the injury had been treated by rest and antiinflammatory agents, only to have the symptoms recur each time normal activities were initiated.

SYMPTOMS OF CARPAL INSTABILITY, DISSOCIATIVE (CID)

The majority of patients with CID complain of pain with activity. They frequently mention popping, catching, and locking of the wrist during sports activity or at their jobs if they frequently flex and extend their wrists in the workplace. Often, they state that the pain is intermittent: as long as they can hold the wrist still, there is no problem, but as soon as the wrist is held in the wrong position and a torque is put on it, they have severe pain. Once they move the wrist back to the former position, the pain goes away. Thus, the pain has a clearly described mechanical component.

PHYSICAL EXAMINATION FOR CID

The clinical test for instability of the scaphoid consists of the examiner's placing a thumb against the distal (palmar) pole of the patient's scaphoid while the wrist is in ulnar deviation. The examiner then brings the wrist into radial deviation and an unstable scaphoid will be forced to sublux dorsally, causing pain at the scapholunate joint and producing a palpable clunk when the scaphoid drops back into the scaphoid fossa of the radius.

Point tenderness is another important physical sign. The scapholunate injury frequently is tender at the site of the 3–4 portal; the lunotriquetral injury is tender at the site of the 6R portal. In another test, the "shuck" test, the examiner holds the radius stable with one hand and carpus stable with the other hand and moves the wrist dorsally and palmarly. Often the patient with gross instability of either the scapholunate or the lunotriquetral joint will have increased mobility in this area as compared to that in the opposite wrist. In order to evaluate the ulnar side of the wrist, the patient's elbow is supported on the examining table, and the examiner places a hand in the patient's hand and compresses the ulnar side of the wrist with dorsiflexion and palmar flexion in addition to ulnar deviation and compression. Frequently, the patient with lunotriquetral instability will then have exquisite pain on the ulnar side of the wrist. It must be remembered that this pain is difficult to distinguish from that caused by a lesion of the triangular fibrocartilage.

ROUTINE ROENTGENOGRAMS

Routine roentgenograms for suspected carpal instability include standard anteroposterior and lateral views, as

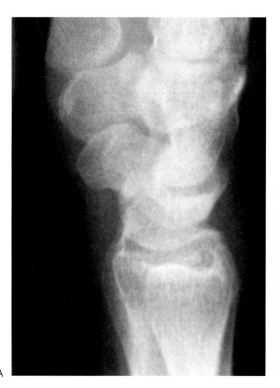 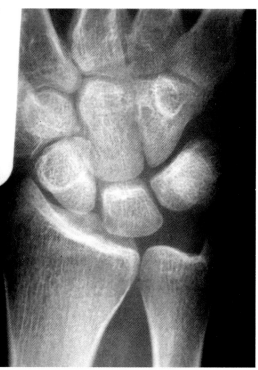

A   B

FIG. 1. A: Lateral view of the wrist reveals a dorsal intercalated segmental instability (DISI) with the lunate tilted dorsally and the scaphoid flexed palmarly. The scapholunate angle is approximately 90°. **B:** AP view of the wrist reveals a ring sign and a foreshortened scaphoid. These indicate palmar flexion of the scaphoid. The lunate is quadrangular in shape, indicating a dorsiflexed position. Despite the absence of a significant gap this roentgenogram is consistent with a scapholunate dissociation.

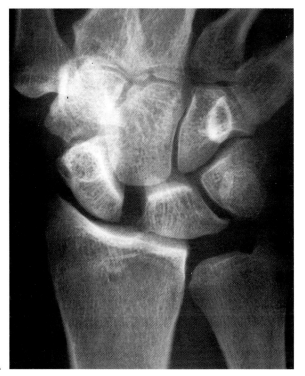
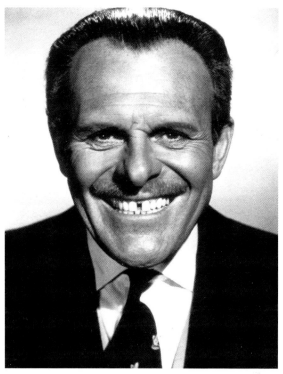

A   B

FIG. 2. **A:** AP view of the wrist demonstrates a foreshortened scaphoid with a ring sign and evidence of palmar flexion. The lunate again is quadrangular and the triquetrum is riding up on the hamate, all indicating a dorsiflexed position. In addition, there is a gap between the scaphoid and the lunate. **B:** A classic gap (actor Terry Thomas).

well as radial and ulnar deviation views. Scapholunate dissociation may be manifested by palmar flexion of the scaphoid with dorsiflexion of the lunate and triquetrum (Fig. 1) or a separation between the scaphoid and the lunate (Fig. 2). The classical sign of a lunotriquetral lesion is dorsiflexion of the triquetrum with volar flexion of the scaphoid and lunate. There may be a separation of the lunate and triquetrum, with a step-off in their normal arc.

SPECIAL STUDIES

Special studies include arthrography, fluoroscopy, and magnetic resonance (MR) imaging. These studies are de-

scribed in detail in the radiology section of this book. Although often unnecessary for diagnosing a tear of the scapholunate or of the lunotriquetral ligament, they may be helpful in questionable cases, and for such cases triple-injection arthrography is recommended.

INCIDENCE OF CARPAL LIGAMENT INJURIES IN AN ARTHROSCOPIC WRIST PRACTICE

In reviewing 82 consecutive patients with wrist injury seen at our institution, we found 44 (54%) to have had some injury to the carpal ligaments (Table 1): 21 partial and 5 complete injuries of the scapholunate; 15 partial

TABLE 1. *Findings in 80 patients undergoing wrist arthroscopy*

Type of injury	No. patients
Interosseous ligamentous injuries	44
Triangular fibrocartilage complex tears	18
Chondromalacia	9
Ganglion cyst	3
Loose bodies	2
Diffuse synovitis	2
Arthrofibrosis	2

TABLE 2. *Type of ligamentous injury sustained based on findings at arthroscopy*

Ligament	Degree of injury		
	Partial	Complete	Total
Scapholunate	21	5	26
Lunotriquetral	15	6	21
Ulnotriquetral	4	7	11
Radioscaphocapitate	1		1
Ulnocarpal	1		1

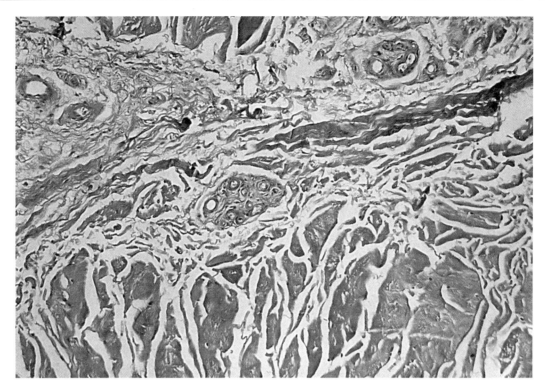

FIG. 3. Histologic section of the dorsal aspect of the scapholunate ligament indicating blood vessels and heavy cross-striations of collagen with histologic evidence of a true ligament. Specimen is 6 mm thick. (Courtesy of Dr. M. Berger.)

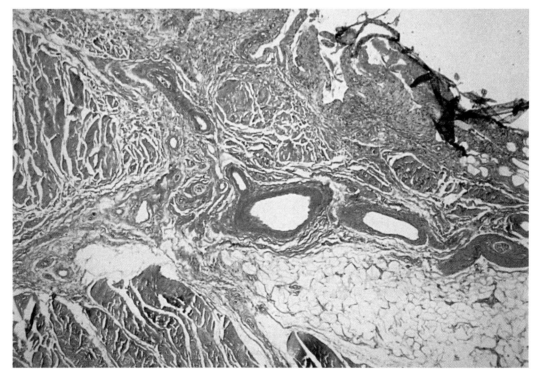

FIG. 4. Histologic section of the palmar aspect of the scapholunate ligament, with evidence of excellent blood supply and moderately heavy collagen fibers. Specimen is about 4 mm thick. (Courtesy of Dr. M. Berger.)

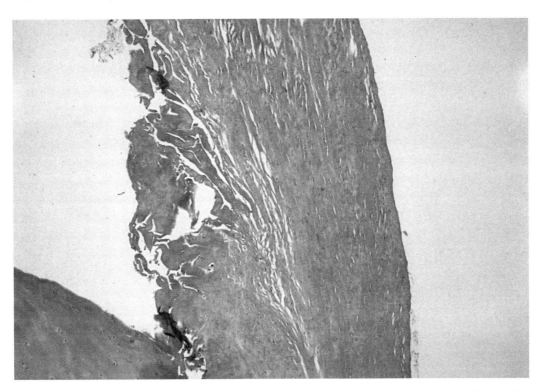

FIG. 5. Histologic section of the midportion of the scapholunate ligament, having no evidence of a synovial lining or of any evidence of any vasculature. Specimen is only 2 mm thick; it was mechanically very weak and primarily fibrocartilage. (Courtesy of Dr. M. Berger.)

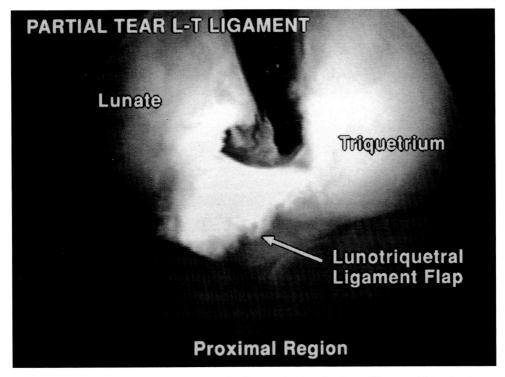

FIG. 6. Partial lunotriquetral ligament tear in the proximal region in an 18-year-old tennis player who had had symptoms for 18 months. Flap resection led to complete resolution of symptoms.

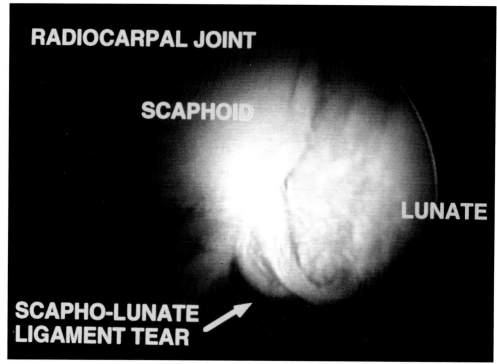

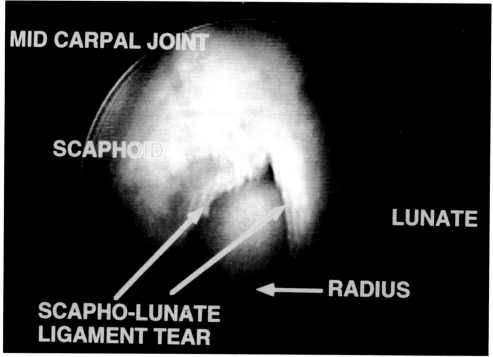

FIG. 7A–E. A: Scapholunate tear from the radiocarpal joint with frayed portion of the scapho-lunate ligament hanging in the radiocarpal joint. **B:** View from the midcarpal joint between the scaphoid and lunate, looking into the scapholunate joint and at the scapholunate ligament tear. The top of this view is palmar.

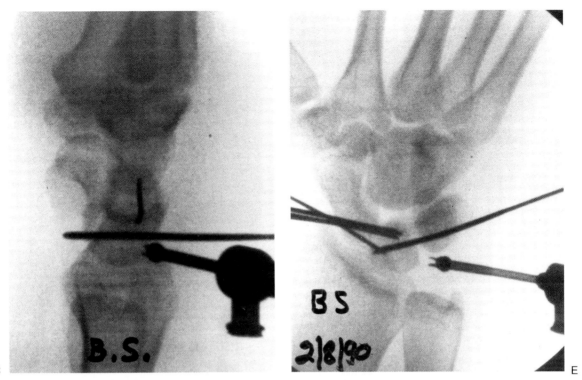

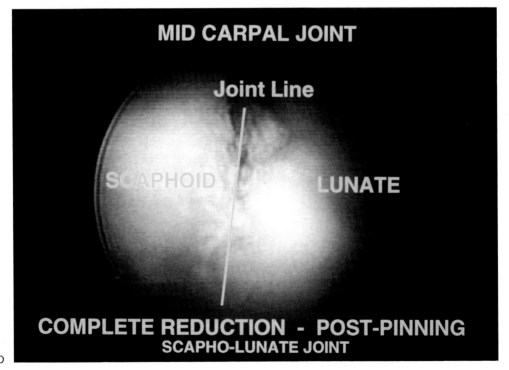

FIG. 7. (*Continued*) **C:** Dorsal-to-palmar pin is placed in the lunate. The second pin is placed in the scaphoid. The pins act as joy sticks to align the scaphonate and lunate. **D:** The joint line is completely reduced while being viewed through the midcarpal joint. **E:** Reduction of the scapholunate joint with pinning. The dorsal-to-palmar lunate pin is removed. The pins are cut off at the level of the skin.

and 6 complete injuries of the lunotriquetral; and 4 partial and 7 complete injuries of the ulnocarpal ligaments (Table 2). Seven patients had multiple-ligament injuries. Arthroscopy has enabled us to recognize that the majority of carpal ligament injuries are partial and that they are a common cause of chronic wrist pain of unknown etiology.

ANATOMY AND MECHANICAL PROPERTIES OF THE INTERCARPAL LIGAMENTS

In 1991, Berger described the anatomy and mechanical properties of the subregions of the intercarpal ligaments (1). He found that there is a true intercapsular ligament in the dorsal region that is about 6 mm thick, has transverse collagen fibers, has a rich blood supply and a synovial lining, and, mechanically, is the most important and the strongest of the intercarpal ligaments (Fig. 3).

The palmar region also is a true ligament, about 4 mm thick. It has oblique collagen fibers, a moderate blood supply, and a synovial lining. However, Berger found that it only resisted a dorsal translation during mechanical testing (Fig. 4) (1).

The proximal region, that is, the area between the dorsal and the palmar intercarpal ligaments, is only about 2 mm thick and is not a true ligament. It is made up of fibrocartilage, has a poor blood supply, does not have a synovial lining, and, mechanically, is extremely weak (Fig. 5).

ARTHROSCOPIC CATEGORIZATION OF INTERCARPAL LIGAMENT INJURIES

Utilizing the information gleaned from the classical descriptions of intercarpal ligament injuries as well as the new information provided by arthroscopy, it can be seen that intercarpal ligament injuries fall into three major groups. Group 1 injuries are partial tears of the scapholunate or lunotriquetral ligaments: they are stable; roentgenograms are normal; and arthrography may or may not be positive.

Group 2 injuries are acute complete scapholunate or lunotriquetral ligament injuries: They are unstable; they invariably involve the dorsal region; and they may involve the proximal and palmar subregions as well. Roentgenographically, they present with dorsal intercalated segmental instability (DISI) or volar intercalated segmental instability (VISI). Usually arthrography will be positive but no degenerative changes will be seen.

Group 3 injuries are chronic complete injuries: they have an unstable pattern like that in group 2, but in addition they have degenerative changes, most classically in the radial styloid and the capitolunate joint.

TREATMENT

Group 1 injuries, or partial tears, involve the proximal subregion of the scapholunate or lunotriquetral joint and are ideally suited for arthroscopic debridement. Injury in this area of the ligament causes no instability; rather, the symptoms are caused by the torn flap of tissue irritating the joint (Fig. 6). Once this flap is debrided, a high percentage of these patients have relief of their symptoms.

For group 2 injuries, the duration from injury to examination usually is 3–6 months; the injuries must be reduced for relief of symptoms. The first step is diagnostic arthroscopy of the radiocarpal joint: the dorsal region is frequently torn and there is instability of the carpal bones between the scaphoid, the lunate (Fig. 7A), and/or the triquetrum. The radiocarpal joint is debrided first; then, if there is still instability (Fig. 7B), the next step is to place a joy stick (a 0.62 K-wire) in the lunate from dorsal to palmar, and then, using a mini C-arm, to place a 0.45 K-wire into the scaphoid (Fig. 7C) in such a way that it will cross the scapholunate ligament as it is advanced. These two wires allow manipulation of both the scaphoid and the lunate. The alignment should be observed on the C-arm first and then checked for anatomic accuracy by viewing it through the midcarpal portal (Fig. 7D). Once anatomic alignment is assured, the scapholunate joint should be pinned with four pins placed across it (Fig. 7E). The wrist then is placed in a compression dressing for 2 days, followed by short-arm casting for 8 weeks. Then the pins are removed and mobilization is begun. The patient is returned to full activity at 4 months.

Long-term follow-up of a large series of this type of repair is not yet available. Although it is used primarily for the treatment of unstable complete scapholunate tears, this repair also has been found to be effective in the treatment of unstable complete lunotriquetral lesions.

Arthroscopy of group 3 tears shows significant degenerative changes and/or an unreducible and fixed deformity. Currently, group 3 tears cannot be treated arthroscopically.

REFERENCES

1. Berger M. Evaluation of the histology and material properties of the subgroup of the scapholunate ligaments. Presented at the 9th Wrist Investigators Workshop, Orlando, FL, October 1991.
2. Dobyns JH, Linscheid RL, Macksoud WS, Seigert JJ. Carpal instability, nondissociative. Presented at the 54th Annual Meeting of the American Academy of Orthopaedic Surgeons, San Francisco, 1987.
3. Linscheid RL, Dobyns JH, Beabout JW, Bryan RS. Traumatic instability of the wrist. Diagnosis, classification and pathomechanics. *J Bone Joint Surg* [Am] 1972;54:1612.
4. Mayfield JK, Johnson RP, Kilcoyne RK. Carpal dislocations: Pathomechanics and progressive perilunar instability. *J Hand Surg* 1980;5:226.
5. Taleisnik J. *The Wrist.* New York: Churchill Livingstone, 1985.

Palmar Midcarpal Instability

David M. Lichtman, M.D., RADM, USN

Instability of the midcarpal joint was first described in 1934 by Mouchet and Belot (7). However, it was not until 1980 that midcarpal instability (MCI) was recognized to be a source of clinical symptoms (5). In 1981 Lichtman and Schneider described a small series of patients who presented with a volar sag at the midcarpal joint and who complained of a spontaneous clunk at the triquetrohamate joint with ulnar deviation of the wrist (6). Anatomic studies at that time revealed that the ulnar arm of the arcuate ligament, also called the volar capitotriquetral ligament, is the primary stabilizer of the midcarpal joint. This ligament inserts proximally on the volar triquetrum, triquetrolunate ligament, and ulnar corner of the lunate. It then runs horizontally to the proximal hamate, to which it sends some fibers, and then inserts distally into the neck of the capitate. Sectioning of this sturdy ligament created midcarpal laxity that resembled the clinical picture of midcarpal instability. A more recent study (4) has shown that in addition to the horizontal fibers of the arcuate ligament, there exist vertical fibers that course from the volar triquetrum to the hook of the hamate and pisohamate ligament. These fibers blend with the fascial insertion of the hypothenar muscles as well as with the insertion of the tendon of the flexor carpi ulnaris around the pisiform. This confluence of structures is called the ulnar arcuate ligament complex (UALC) (Fig. 1).

Laxity of the UALC permits the head of the capitate and proximal hamate to sag volarly from their "nested" positions in the midcarpal joint. This volar subluxation induces a passive volar intercalary segmental instability (VISI) pattern or volar flexion deformity of the entire proximal row (Fig. 2). From this position the normal articular interactions of the midcarpal joint cannot occur, i.e., with radial to ulnar deviation the normal smooth transition from proximal row flexion to proximal row extension will not be seen. Instead, the VISI pattern persists until almost complete ulnar deviation, at which time a rapid "catch-up clunk" occurs as the proximal row jumps from excessive flexion into physiologic exten-

sion, and the head of the capitate and the hamate suddenly reduce themselves.

In 1990 Viegas demonstrated that the dorsal radiolunotriquetral ligament also plays a major role in stabilizing the proximal row (8). Following division of this ligament a VISI deformity occurs which results in the same kinematic abnormality as described above. What I have presented thus far is palmar midcarpal instability (PMCI) and is, by far, the most common clinical type of MCI. A few cases of dorsal MCI have also been seen, but this condition is very rare. Combined dorsal and palmar MCI may also exist. Other authors have referred to instabilities at the midcarpal joint as the chronic capitolunate instability (CLIP) (2) and carpal instability, nondissociative (CIND) syndromes (1), but we believe these terms are less descriptive names for essentially the same clinical condition as described above.

Recent unpublished clinical and laboratory investigations have shown that external dorsally directed pressure on the pisiform bone can eliminate the clunk of PMCI by reducing the proximal row VISI deformity and distal row sag. This occurs because the pisiform and its triquetral articulation are distal to the axis of rotation of the proximal row in the transverse plane. Thus, upward pressure on the pisiform causes a downward rotation of the lunate and triquetrum—out of its subluxed VISI position. Direct observation has also shown that active contraction of the extensor carpi ulnaris (ECU), flexor carpi ulnaris (FCU), and hypothenar muscles can reduce the sagging (VISI) midcarpal joint. Some patients with MCI can eliminate the clunk by contracting these muscles prior to ulnar deviation of the wrist. More investigation needs to be done to determine the role of passive splinting as well as muscle rehabilitation in treating milder cases of PMCI.

The diagnosis of PMCI can be made easily by history and physical examination once the examiner has had previous experience with this condition. The volar wrist sag can be seen by carefully looking at the wrist's configuration (Fig. 3). The "clunk" with ulnar deviation is

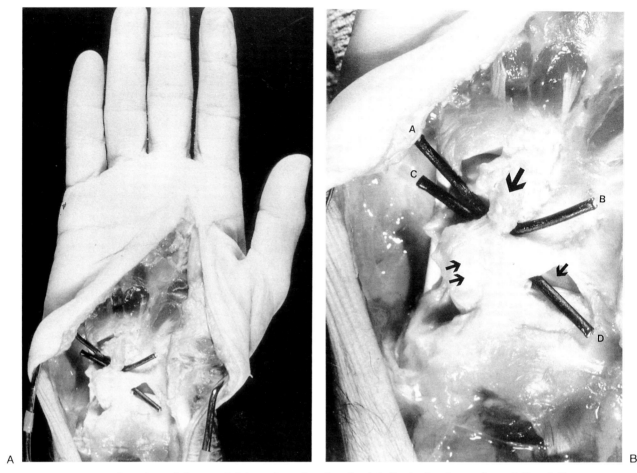

FIG. 1. A: Overview of dissected right cadaver hand and wrist. Contents of carpal canal, the pisiform bone, and pisohamate ligament have been removed. The radiolunate and radioscapholunate ligaments have also been removed to help visualization of ulnar arcuate ligament complex. **B:** Closeup view of the same wrist. Large arrow points to hook of hamate; small arrow to head of capitate in space of Poirier; double arrow points to triquetral facet of pisotriquetral joint. Stick A–B runs beneath vertical fibers of ulnar arcuate ligament. Stick C–D runs under vertical fibers distally and broader horizontal fibers of arcuate ligament proximally.

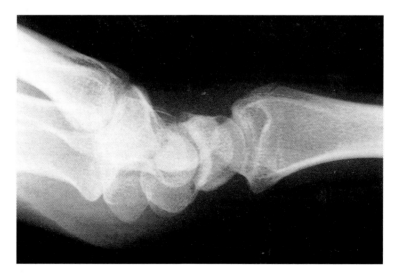

FIG. 2. Lateral radiograph with the wrist in neutral deviation demonstrates the VISI deformity of the entire proximal row with volar positioning of the head of the capitate.

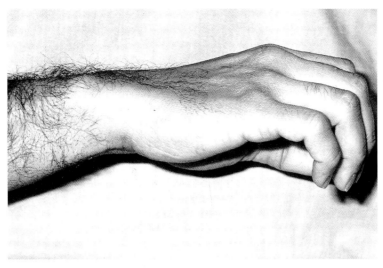

FIG. 3. Volar wrist sag seen best from the ulnar side during clinical examination.

obvious as the midpalmar sag reduces itself spontaneously. This reduction can be reproduced passively by the examiner by gentle axial compression, ulnar deviation, and intercarpal supination. The patient will tell you that this maneuver exactly duplicates the symptoms.

Radiographic and arthroscopic studies are essential to confirm the diagnosis. Aside from the characteristic VISI deformity and volar sag at the midcarpal joint (Fig. 2), the plane films are essentially normal. Because the subluxation is easily reducible, the plane films may not show the defect. In a few of our cases a dissociative lesion of the proximal row has coexisted with the PMCI. In these cases, the x-ray picture can confuse the diagnosis, because the signs and symptoms of PMCI almost always overshadow those of dissociative lesions, yet dissociative lesions of the proximal row are more striking on the x-ray films.

Video fluoroscopy will always confirm the diagnosis of PMCI if you know what to look for. The sudden transition of the proximal row from VISI to DISI as the wrist goes into ulnar deviation will be seen to be the source of the clunk. The entire proximal row will rotate as a unit distinguishing PMCI from triquetrolunate (TL) and/or scapholunate (SL) instability. When these dissociative lesions coexist with PMCI, the individual components can be identified, but it takes practice and patience to sort them out while viewing the videos.

Wrist arthroscopy is an important diagnostic adjunct to video fluoroscopy. It is essential to rule out dissociative lesions prior to surgical treatment of MCI. Gross TL or SL instability will compromise the surgical results of MCI repairs. Even mild dissociative lesions can be aggravated by procedures that stabilize the midcarpal joint. Although arthrography can also give accurate information on dissociative wrist lesions, this procedure is not as sensitive as arthroscopy. Bone scans do not add specific

diagnostic information, and the indications for magnetic resonance imaging have not been fully defined for carpal instabilities.

Our treatment of PMCI started with ligamentous stabilization of the triquetrohamate joint and then evolved to limited arthrodesis of the midcarpal joint (triquetrohamate or triquetrohamate–lunate–capitate fusion). Most recently we have taken advantage of our new understanding of midcarpal anatomy to perform what we feel is a more physiologic reconstruction—advancement and tightening of the UALC and reefing of the volar capsular ligaments. Through an extended carpal tunnel approach we identify and advance the distal insertion of the sturdy horizontal fibers of the UALC. Care must be taken to free its fibrous insertions into the volar surfaces of the hamate and capitate. The proximal insertion into the triquetrum, volar triquetrolunate ligament, and lunate is left intact. Pulling this dissected ligament in a volar direction and advancing it distally corrects the VISI deformity of the proximal row (Fig. 4A, B). Distal advancement on the capitate tightens the complex and prevents recurrence of the volar sag. The advanced ligament is secured by heavy sutures passed through drill holes from volar to dorsal and tied over the dorsal neck of the capitate. Next, the entire volar capsule is reefed by placing heavy sutures between the radioscaphocapitate and the radiolunotriquetral ligaments, eliminating the space of Poirier. The proximal row is then secured to the distal row with K-wires in the neutral position. Next, through a separate dorsal incision the dorsal radiolunotriquetral ligaments are advanced or reefed (Fig. 4C). The K-wires are left in place for 10 to 12 weeks. Range of motion of the wrist is not attempted until 12 weeks postoperatively and is intentionally regained slowly over the next 3 months.

In a recently published review of our first 16 operative

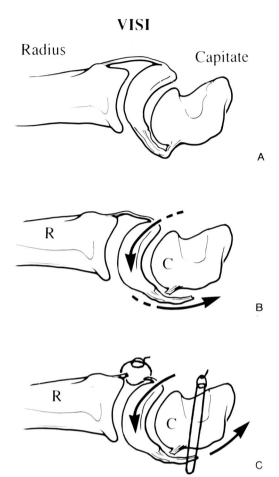

VISI

Radius   Capitate

A

R   C

B

R   C

C

FIG. 4. A: Schematic representation of the lax ulnar arcuate ligament with proximal attachment to the lunate and triquetrum and distal attachment to capitate. Note VISI position of lunate in drawing. **B:** Schematic drawing of advancement of the distal attachment of the arcuate ligament. Note the proximal row as represented by the lunate being drawn out of VISI into neutral alignment. This advancement can be done by reefing or by actual division and resuture of the distal insertion of the horizontal fibers of the ulnar arcuate ligament. **C:** Dorsal and palmar radiocarpal ligaments tightened to stabilize proximal row.

cases, it was clear that midcarpal arthrodesis was the most reliable operative procedure, as 100% of patients treated with fusion obtained a satisfactory result. Nevertheless, when given a choice, many patients choose a soft tissue reconstruction knowing that if the clunk recurs a

fusion can be done at a later date. Future research in the area of MCI will revolve around newer methods of treatment. We are excited about the prospect of splinting and muscle retraining techniques for milder cases. For resistant cases surgical therapy is currently the only option. It seems inevitable that arthroscopic reconstruction of the UALC will eventually replace or enhance the current open advancement technique of the UALC.

In summary, palmar midcarpal instability is an uncommon but not rare clinical condition. Recent improved understanding of the anatomy and physiology of the midcarpal joint has led to the development of promising new rehabilitative as well as operative techniques. Arthroscopic examination of the wrist is helpful in ruling out dissociative lesions of the proximal row, which, if they exist, must be addressed prior to or concomitant with the surgical treatment of PMCI. It is anticipated that innovative techniques for arthroscopic repair of the ulnar arcuate ligament complex will eventually be developed.

Disclaimer. The opinions and/or assertions contained in this chapter are the private views of the author and are not to be construed as reflecting the official policy or position of the United States Navy, Department of Defense, or the United States Government.

REFERENCES

1. Dobyns JH, Linscheid RL, Wadih SM, et al. Carpal instability, non-dissociative (CIND). Presented at the Annual Meeting of the American Academy of Orthopaedic Surgeons, San Francisco, Jan. 1987.
2. Johnson RP, Carrera GF. Chronic capitolunate instability. *J Bone Joint Surg* 1980;68A:1164–1176.
3. Lichtman DM, Bruckner JD, Culp RW, Alexander CE. Palmer midcarpal instability: results of surgical reconstruction. *J Hand Surg* 1993;18;(2):307–315.
4. Lichtman DM, Niccolai TA, et al. The ulnar arcuate ligament complex, its anatomy and functional significance. Presented at the 43rd Annual Meeting of the American Society for Surgery of the Hand, Baltimore, Sept. 14–17, 1988.
5. Lichtman DM, Schneider JR, Swafford AR. Midcarpal instability. Presented at the 35th Annual Meeting of the Am Soc for Surg of the Hand, Atlanta, Feb. 4–6, 1980.
6. Lichtman DM, Schneider JR, Swafford AR, et al. Ulnar midcarpal instability. Clinical and laboratory analysis. *J Hand Surg* 1981;6:515–523.
7. Mouchet A, Belot J. Poignet a resault (subluxation mediocarpienne en avant). *Bull Mem Soc Natl Chir* 1934;60:1243–1244.
8. Viegas SF, Pogue DJ, Hokanson JA. Ulnar-sided perilunate instability: an anatomic and biomechanic study. *J Hand Surg* 1990;15A:268–277.

Triangular Fibrocartilage Complex

Diagnostic and Operative Arthroscopy

Gary G. Poehling, M.D., *L. Andrew Koman*, M.D., *David B. Siegel*, M.D.,
and David S. Ruch, M.D.

Although considerable controversy exists concerning the role of the triangular fibrocartilage (TFC) as a potential cause of pain on the ulnar side of the wrist (1,3,4,9–11), injuries to the TFC and the ulnocarpal ligaments are considerably more common than other intraarticular causes of ulnar-sided wrist pain (5,8). A thorough understanding of the anatomic components of the triangular fibrocartilage complex (TFCC) is necessary in evaluating and treating ulnar-sided wrist pain. This chapter reviews the normal anatomy and histology, pathologic changes with their classification, and diagnostic as well as operative arthroscopic treatment of lesions of the TFCC.

ANATOMY

The TFCC originates at the sigmoid notch of the distal radius immediately distal to the articular surface of the distal radioulnar joint. Short, thick collagen bundles project 1–2 mm from the radius into the TFCC (Fig. 1A and B) (2). The articular disc inserts firmly into bone at the base of the ulnar styloid process (Fig. 2A and B). The central portion of the articular disc is poorly vascularized, whereas the peripheral portion is well vascularized (Fig. 3A–C). The articular disc is reinforced by the dorsal and palmar distal radioulnar ligaments, which blend smoothly with the disc (Fig. 4A and B) and provide stability to the distal radioulnar joint. Palmarly, the ulnolunate and ulnotriquetral ligaments are attached firmly to the palmar radioulnar ligament (Fig. 5), and the dorsal wrist capsule attaches to the dorsal distal radioulnar ligament.

In summary, the peripheral attachments of the TFCC are thick, strong, and well perfused, whereas the central articular disc is relatively thin and has no demonstrable blood supply. The improved healing capacity following injury to the peripheral portions of the TFCC may be related to the blood supply in this area.

ANATOMIC CLASSIFICATION OF LESIONS OF THE TRIANGULAR CARTILAGE COMPLEX

Palmer classified lesions of the TFCC into two broad categories—traumatic (type I) and degenerative (type II)—based on the arthroscopic appearance and location of the lesions (2,6) (Table 1).

Traumatic Lesions

Palmer described four types of traumatic tears of the TFCC.

Type IA is a horizontal tear in the articular disc. These tears are linear from dorsal to palmar and adjacent to the sigmoid notch of the distal radius (Fig. 6). They are thought to be the most common type of traumatic injury to the TFCC, and frequently result from a hyperextension injury or a twisting injury of the wrist with impact loading.

Type IB is a peripheral detachment or avulsion of the insertion of the TFCC at the base of the ulnar styloid

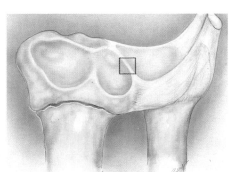

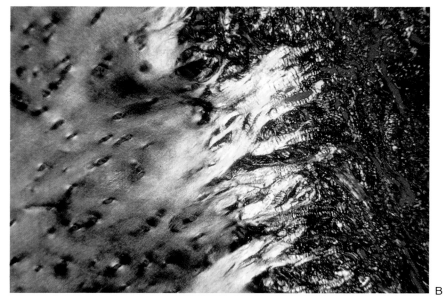

CHAPTER 8

A   B

FIG. 1. A: Outlined area of histologic section represents the origin of the articular disc from the radius. **B:** Transverse histologic section of the radial origin of the articular disc. Short, thick fibers extend from the radius (*left*) side into the articular disc (*right*). (×16, polarized light). (From Chidgey, ref. 2, with permission.)

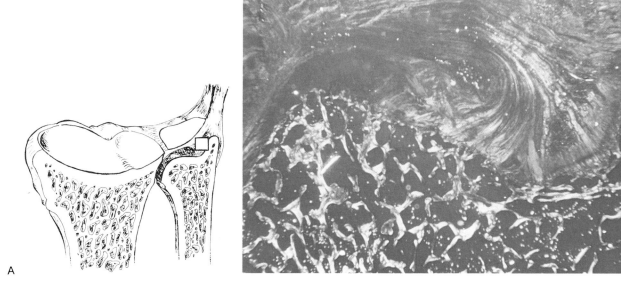

A   B

FIG. 2. A: Outlined area of histologic section represents the ulnar insertion of the articular disc. **B:** Collagen fibers in the lower portion of the articular disc turn proximally and radially to insert on the ulnar head. The collagen fibers in the upper portion of the articular disc surround the base of the ulnar styloid. (×2.5, polarized light). (From Chidgey, ref. 2, with permission.)

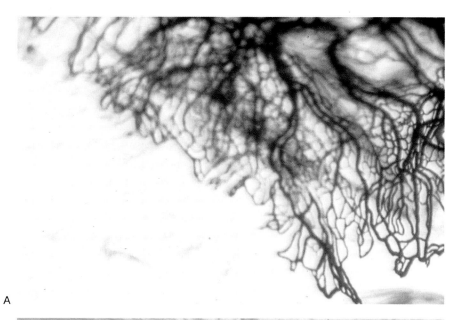

A

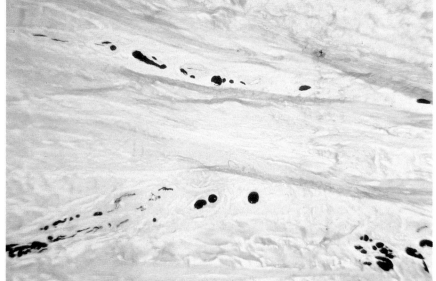

B

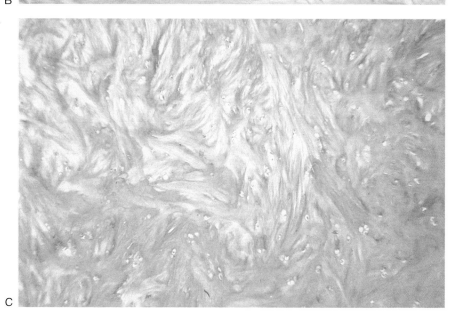

C

FIG. 3. A: The vessels in the peripheral 20% of the articular disc form arcades. These vessels are more dense along the more ulnar aspect of the articular disc where this section was made. **B:** The radioulnar ligaments and peripheral 15% to 20% of the articular disc demonstrate good vascularity after vessels are filled with India ink. This section is the dorsal radioulnar ligament. **C:** No vessels have been identified in the central area of the articular disc after India ink vascular injection. (From Chidgey, ref. 2, with permission.)

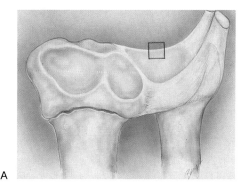

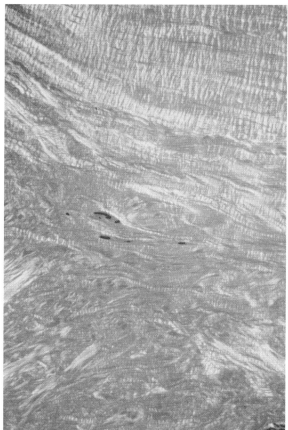

FIG. 4. A: Outlined area of histologic section represents the junction between the dorsal radioulnar ligament and the articular disc. **B:** Transverse histologic section of the junction between the dorsal radioulnar ligament (*top*) and the articular disc (*bottom*). (×16, polarized light). (From Chidgey, ref. 2, with permission.)

(Fig. 7). This type of injury may be associated with distal radius fractures or with other injuries to the upper extremity that are remote from the TFCC itself.

Type IC involves tears of the ulnocarpal ligaments (ulnolunate and ulnotriquetral) and is usually caused by a direct fall on the ulnar side of the hand (Fig. 8).

Type ID is a complete detachment of the radial origin of the TFCC from the sigmoid notch of the distal radius (Fig. 9). A portion of bone is attached to the TFCC. Usually this lesion is associated with instability of the distal radioulnar joint and is caused by a severe impact or twisting injury of the wrist and forearm.

Most patients with traumatic lesions of the TFCC describe pain on the ulnar side of the wrist, which is exacerbated with any activity that requires forearm rotation. Weakness, catching, and snapping also are noted. Although the pain may improve with rest, symptoms frequently are exacerbated once activities are resumed.

Physical examination often demonstrates tenderness over the dorsum of the TFC. The stability of the distal radioulnar joint should be assessed through a full range of forearm rotation. The ulnar impaction sign should be checked. In this test the examiner stabilizes the forearm

(Fig. 10) and then brings the wrist into maximal dorsiflexion and ulnar deviation, thus impacting the ulnar carpus against the distal ulna and the TFC. In patients with tears of the TFC and associated synovitis on the ulnar side of the wrist, this maneuver commonly causes immediate pain. The amount of dorsal–palmar translation of the ulnar carpus should be compared with that of the normal wrist, and the stability of the distal radioulnar joint should be noted.

Radiographic examination should include plain and stress radiographs. In patients with types IA and ID lesions, triple-injection arthrograms demonstrate dye leaking from the radiocarpal joint to the distal radioulnar joint through the radial side of the TFC; in patients with type IB lesions, pooling of dye at the base of the ulnar styloid process is characteristic, although a communication between the radiocarpal and the distal radioulnar joints may be noted. Type IC lesions may be associated with instability of the distal ulna, and radiocarpal arthrography may demonstrate communication between the radiocarpal and midcarpal joints. These findings may cause type IC lesions to be mistaken for tears of the lunotriquetral ligament.

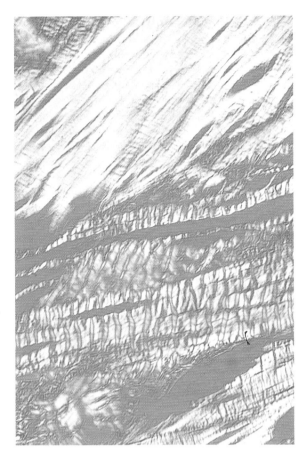

FIG. 5. Fibers of the palmar ulnocarpal ligament (*top*) interdigitate with the palmar radioulnar ligament (*bottom*). (×16, polarized light). (From Chidgey, ref. 2, with permission.)

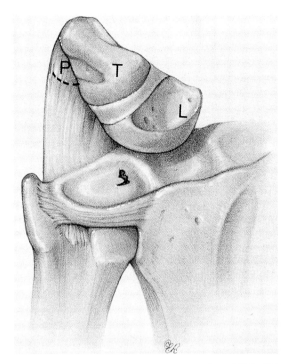

FIG. 6. Palmar type IA traumatic tear of the TFC. This is the most common tear seen; there is usually a small flap that is unstable. Removal of the flap usually relieves the patient's symptoms. P, pisiform; T, triquetrum; L, lunate. (Illustration by Elizabeth Roselius, © 1993. From Green, ref. 10, with permission.)

TABLE 1. *Palmer's classification of TFCC tears*

Type I—Traumatic
  A. Horizontal tear adjacent to the radius
  B. Peripheral detachment from ulna
  C. Tear of the ulnocarpal ligaments
  D. Avulsion of the radius
Type II—Degenerative
  A. Thinning of the articular disc
  B. Thinning of the articular disc and chondromalacia
  C. Tear of the articular disc and chondromalacia
  D. Tear of the articular disc, chondromalacia, and partial tearing of the lunotriquetral ligament
  E. Tear of the articular disc, chondromalacia, tear of the lunotriquetral ligament, and arthritis of the radioulnar joint

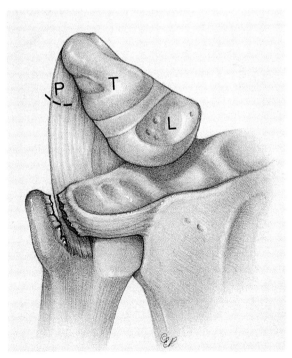

FIG. 7. Palmar type IB traumatic TFC tear. This demonstrates an avulsion of the ulna. This may or may not include a fracture of the ulnar styloid. The resulting loss of tension in the TFC may cause ulnar side symptoms. (Illustration by Elizabeth Roselius, © 1993. From Green, ref. 10, with permission.)

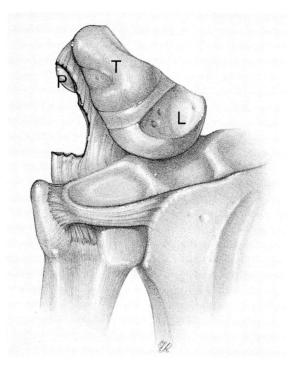

FIG. 8. Palmar type IC traumatic TFC tear is a tear of the ulnocarpal ligament complex, which exposes the pisiform. (Illustration by Elizabeth Roselius, © 1993. From Green, ref. 10, with permission.)

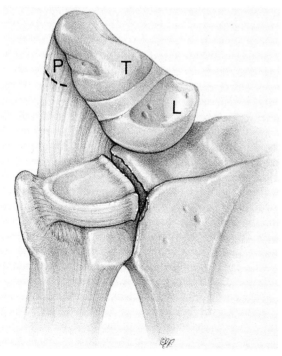

FIG. 9. Palmar type ID traumatic TFC tear is an avulsion of the ulnar border of the sigmoid notch. In acute fractures, these frequently heal, as there are bony edges present on both sides of the avulsion. (Illustration by Elizabeth Roselius, © 1993. From Green, ref. 10, with permission.)

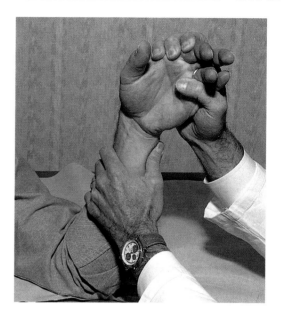

FIG. 10. Ulnar impaction sign photo.

DIAGNOSTIC AND OPERATIVE ARTHROSCOPY

Arthroscopy of the wrist is indicated for the patient who, by history, physical examination, and radiography, has a mechanical disruption of the TFCC. The average patient would have a history of some trauma to the wrist, which when treated by rest becomes painless, but the patient has pain, popping, and catching on the ulnar side with activity. In addition, the injury presents as a diagnostic dilemma or has failed to respond to conservative management consisting of splinting and a period of nonsteroidal antiinflammatory medication. As a diagnostic study, arthroscopy provides additional information regarding the pathoanatomy of the TFCC as well as the remainder of the radiocarpal and midcarpal joints so that subsequent treatment can be based on an improved understanding of the lesion.

Diagnostic arthroscopy is accomplished using standard traction apparatus. The 3–4, 4–5, and 6R portals are used routinely for complete visualization and probing of the TFCC and the lunotriquetral and scapholunate ligaments, as well as the articular surfaces of the lunate, the triquetrum, and the distal radius.

The telescope is placed initially into the 3–4 portal with the probe in the 4–5 portal and the outflow and pressure monitoring system in the 6R portal. Once the diagnosis of a type IA TFCC tear (Fig. 6) is established by direct visualization, the probe is used to assess the stability of the tear. Debridement of the unstable portion of the TFCC is accomplished with 2.9-mm basket forceps or suction basket forceps, as well as with grasping forceps and a motorized shaver. We prefer to use a 3.0-mm, full-

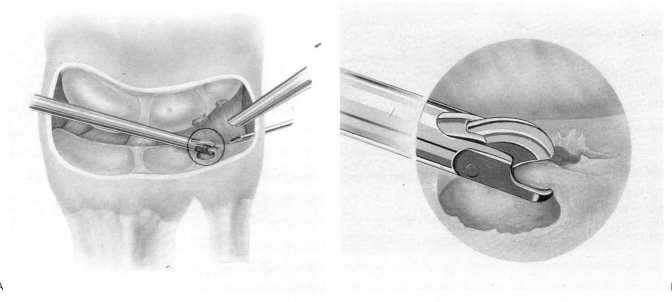

A   B

FIG. 11. **A:** Telescope visualizes the TFCC tear through the 4–5 portal with the suction basket forceps in the 3–4 portal. **B:** Closeup of the suction basket forceps. The tissue is pulled into the jaws of the instrument, which allows easy cutting and removal of the loose portions of the TFCC.

radius, motorized suction shaving device placed into the 4–5 portal with the telescope placed into the 3–4 portal. The rough edges of the tear are debrided with the suction shaving device. A suction basket forceps is then inserted into the 4–5 portal and the loose palmar and radial aspects of the tear are trimmed back to stable tissue. The telescope is then removed from the 3–4 portal and inserted into the 4–5 portal and the suction basket forceps is inserted into the 3–4 portal so that the dorsal and ulnar portions of the tear can be debrided (Fig. 11A and B). The final debridement is accomplished with the motorized shaver so that no rough edges of the TFCC remain. Postoperatively, a wrist splint is applied for 2 days, and active exercises are initiated thereafter. Symptomatic relief and restoration of motion can be expected within 6–12 weeks after surgery. Rarely have we found it necessary to reoperate on these wrists, although occasionally a second tear will develop in a previously debrided area. This tear responds well to repeat debridement.

Type IB lesions (Fig. 7) are associated with extensive synovitis on the ulnar side of the wrist, which requires debridement for complete visualization. The radial, central, dorsal, and palmar aspects of the articular disc appear normal. With the telescope in the 3–4 portal, the probe in the 4–5 portal, and the outflow cannula and pressure monitoring system in the 6R portal, any loss of normal tension in the articular disc suggests a peripheral tear of the TFC as it inserts into the capsule and the base of the ulnar styloid. Because the blood supply in this area of the TFCC is excellent, we recommend repair of this lesion using an arthroscopically assisted suture tech-

nique. The shaver is placed into the 6R portal and the margins of the articular disc are trimmed, as is the adjacent surface of the dorsal capsule (Fig. 12). An incision 1 to 1.5 cm long is made directly over the extensor carpi ulnaris tendon, and the dorsal sheath of the tendon is incised longitudinally. The tendon is retracted to expose

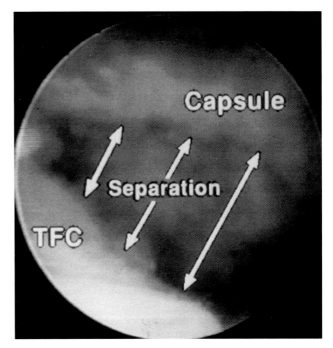

FIG. 12. The ulnar aspect of the TFCC and the capsule are debrided of synovitis, which exposes a wide separation as well as a loss in tightness of the articular disc.

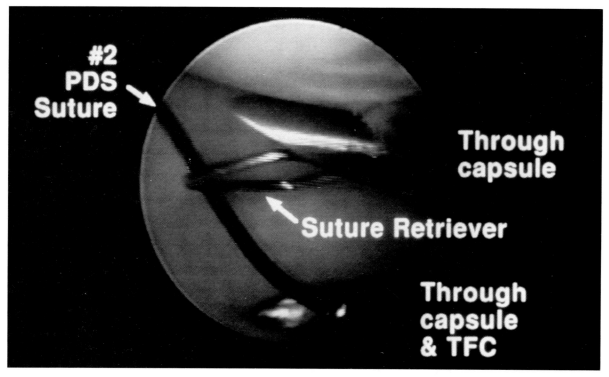

A

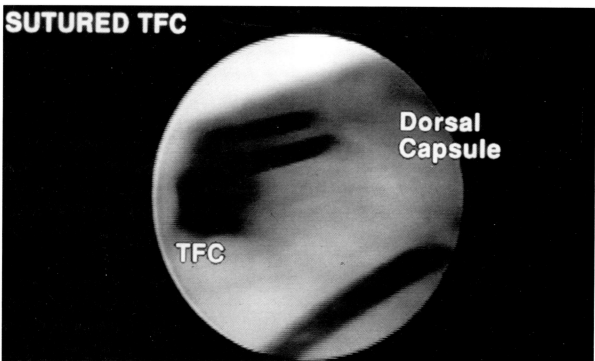

B

FIG. 13. A: The suture passer is proximal and goes through the capsule and the articular disc, while the suture retriever is distal and goes only through the capsule. **B:** In this case, three sutures firmly secure the dorsal capsule and the TFCC.

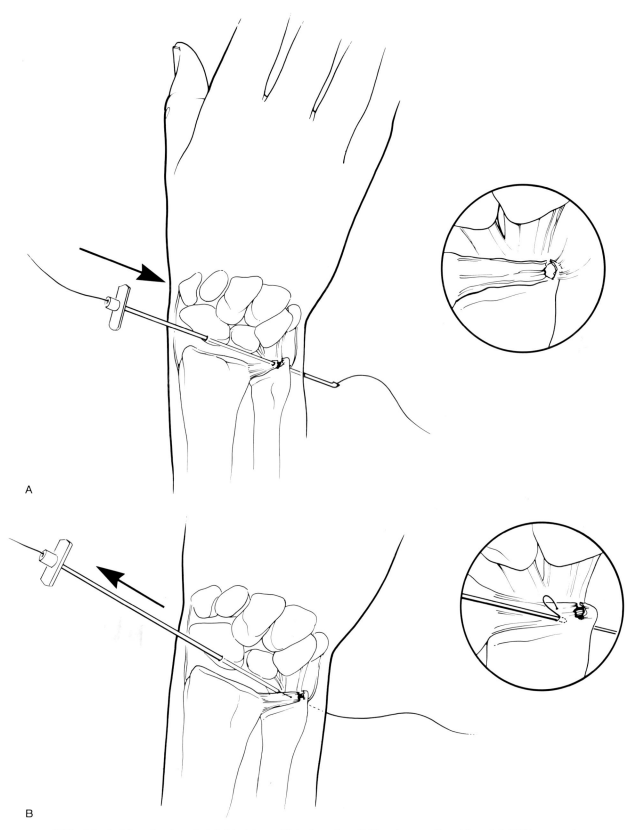

FIG. 14. A: Visualized and debrided type IC lesion. (Inset) Toughy needle with a 2-0 PDS suture is placed. **B:** The needle is withdrawn into the joint, while both ends of the suture are held outside the skin. (Inset) Toughy needle is moved dorsally and reinserted.

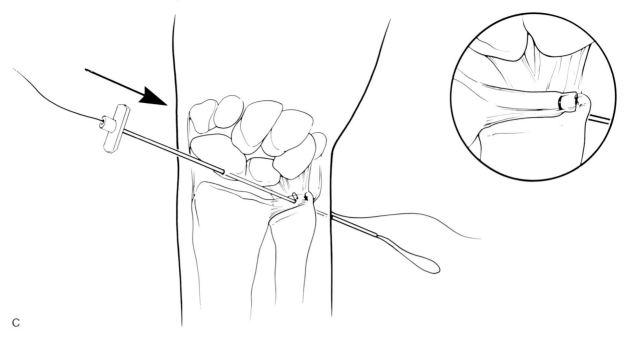

C

FIG. 14. (*Continued*) **C:** Needle is placed through the skin with the suture adjacent to the needle as well as through the needle. (**Inset**) Suture is pulled through the needle and then the needle is removed, leaving a horizontal mattress stitch.

the intratendinous retinaculum. A cannulated needle then is passed through the dorsal capsule and extensor retinaculum into the articular disc 1 to 2 mm from the torn edge of the TFCC. A wire-loop suture retriever is passed similarly through the capsule, and the suture is passed through the cannulated needle and pulled out with the wire-loop suture retriever (Fig. 13A). The articular disc then is tied down to the dorsal capsule and extensor retinaculum (Fig. 13B). As many sutures as necessary to stabilize the TFCC are placed, the number being determined by direct visualization through the telescope in the 4–5 portal.

An alternative method of repairing a type IB lesion is to use a Toughy 20-gauge needle. This is the typical needle used by anesthesiologists to thread an epidural catheter. The telescope is placed in the 4–5 portal and the tear is visualized. The empty needle is inserted into the 1–2 portal and pushed through the periphery of the tear in the TFCC and then through the capsule and skin on the ulnar wrist. A 2-0 PDS suture is then threaded through the needle (Fig. 14A); the needle tip is withdrawn into the joint to be reinserted 5 to 10 mm away from the first needle puncture; and the needle is again pushed through the articular disc, capsule, and skin (Fig. 14B). The suture is then pulled out of the tip of the needle and the needle is withdrawn (Fig. 14C). This leaves a horizontal mattress suture through the torn TFCC. A 1- to 2-cm longitudinal incision is made between the sutures, so that the capsule can be visualized, and the sutures are brought into the wound and tied over the capsule, with care being

taken not to entrap the ulnar sensory nerve. This maneuver firmly approximates the ulnar border of the TFCC and the capsule.

Type IC lesions (Fig. 8) are treated with debridement of the free ligamentous tissue to prevent impingement and interference in the normal gliding of the wrist joint. Most of these tears are partial, and they maintain sufficient stability so that a subsequent reconstruction is not necessary. We have found that most patients have excellent symptomatic relief with debridement alone if a TFCC tear is their only intraarticular problem.

Type ID lesions (Fig. 9) are uncommon and are treated similarly to type IA lesions. Debridement of the unstable edge usually leads to a stable, painless joint.

Degenerative Lesions

Palmer described five types of type II (degenerative) lesions, all believed to be related to the ulnocarpal impingement syndrome (Table 1) (6,7). Type IIA is the earliest stage of ulnocarpal abutment and is characterized by thinning of the articular disc without frank perforation. In type IIB, there is thinning of the articular disc with changes in the hyaline cartilage consistent with chondromalacia on the adjacent surfaces of the ulnar head and lunate. Perforation of the articular disc with chondromalacia on the ulnar head and lunate is seen in type IIC. With progression to type IID lesions, there is partial tearing of the lunotriquetral ligament, further de-

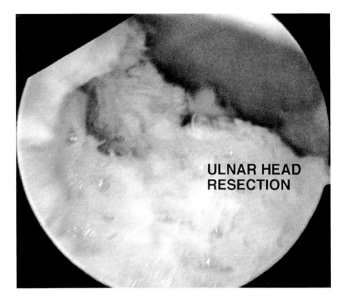

FIG. 15. Ulnar impaction syndrome may be relieved by resecting a small portion of the ulnar head.

struction of articular cartilage, and subchondral bone changes. These lesions immediately precede the more severe degeneration of the articular surfaces characteristic of type IIE lesions. In type IIE lesions, there is fibrillation and fissuring of the articular surfaces of the radioulnar joint, with disruption of the articular disc and the lunotriquetral ligament as well as synovitis. Degenerative lesions almost always occur in the centrum of the articular disc, are usually round with rough edges, and appear to result from impaction of the ulnar carpus on the ulnar head.

Arthroscopic treatment includes debridement of the unstable portion of the degenerated articular disc with intraarticular resection of the ulnar head (the wafer procedure) and debridement of the unstable portion of the lunotriquetral ligament tear. With the telescope in the 3–4 portal, the 2.9-mm shaver in the 4–5 portal, and the outflow and pressure monitoring system in the 6R portal, the unstable portion of the TFCC is debrided in patients with stage IIA or IIB lesions. With stage IIC lesions, debridement of associated flap tears of the articular surface may be necessary as well. The adjacent articular surfaces of the lunate, the triquetrum, and the ulnar head are examined carefully (Fig. 15), and the wrist is stressed into ulnar deviation to assess any impingement of the ulnar carpus on the distal ulna. The information obtained during arthroscopy is correlated with the preoperative clinical evaluation to determine whether resection of the ulnar head is warranted (Fig. 16).

Debridement of the articular disc is necessary for complete visualization before the ulnar head is resected. The ulnar head resection is accomplished with the telescope in the 3–4 portal and a 2.9-mm motorized abrader in the 4–5 portal. The distal 2–3 mm of ulnar head, including the articular cartilage and subchondral bone, is removed under direct visualization. It is necessary to rotate the forearm fully in order to expose the entire ulnar head

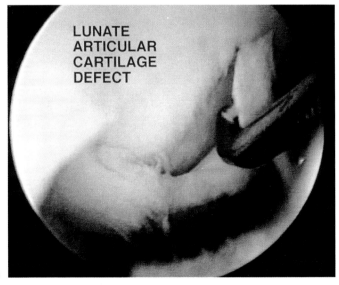

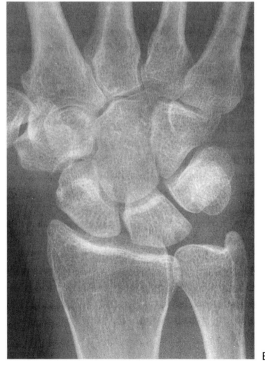

A   B

FIG. 16. A: The ulnar head shows through the TFCC tear with evidence of chondromalacia on the lunate.
B: Radiograph of same patient with impaction of the ulna on the lunate with a lesion on the lunate.

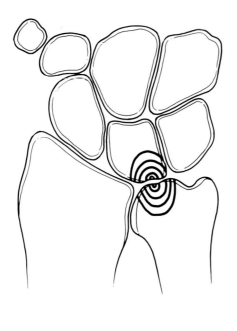

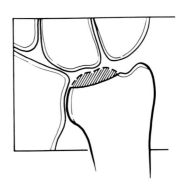

FIG. 17. Resection of the distal 2–3 mm of the ulna effectively decompresses the ulnolunate impingements while preserving radioulnar stability.

through the TFC tear. The articular cartilage of the distal radioulnar joint is left intact to preserve normal forearm rotation (Fig. 17). Copious irrigation is necessary to ensure evacuation of all osseous and cartilaginous debris. (We also have found arthroscopy to be of benefit in assessing the adequacy of resection following the open wafer procedure or in assessing ulnocarpal impingement following diaphyseal ulnar shortening procedures.)

Frequently, type IID lesions are associated with instability of the lunotriquetral joint. It is necessary to insert a probe into the 3–4 portal with the telescope in the 4–5 portal to assess the stability of this joint. The probe is inserted into the articulation in an attempt to separate the two bones. In addition, manual stressing of the lunotriquetral joint is done under direct visualization in order to assess dorsal palmar stability. If the joint appears stable but there is a partial tear, debridement is carried out with a power shaver in the 3–4 portal with the telescope in the 4–5 portal. If, however, instability is noted, then all loose, unstable tissue is debrided back to bleeding tissue. Then, the lunotriquetral joint is reduced under direct visualization and pinned percutaneously, with radiographic guidance for placement of the pins. Radiocarpal, as well as midcarpal, arthroscopy is necessary in order to ensure anatomic alignment of the lunotriquetral joint. These patients also often require debridement of the articular disc and ulnar shortening, as previously described.

Patients with stage IIE lesions do not respond well to debridement procedures because advanced arthritis currently is not amenable to arthroscopically assisted treatment.

REFERENCES

1. Brown DE, Lichtman DM. The evaluation of chronic wrist pain. *Orthop Clin North Am* 1984;15(2):183–192.
2. Chidgey LK. Histologic anatomy of the triangular fibrocartilage. *Hand Clin* 1991;7:249–262.
3. Green DP. The sore wrist without a fracture. *Instr Course Lect* 1985;34:300–313.
4. Menon J, Wood VE, Schoene HR, Frykman GK, Hohl JC, Bestard EA. Isolated tears of the triangular fibrocartilage of the wrist: Results of partial excision. *J Hand Surg* 1984;9A:527–530.
5. Palmer AK. The distal radioulnar joint. Anatomy, biomechanics, and triangular fibrocartilage complex abnormalities. *Hand Clin* 1987;3:31–40.
6. Palmer AK. Triangular fibrocartilage complex lesions: A classification. *J Hand Surg* 1989;14A:594–606.
7. Palmer AK. Triangular fibrocartilage disorders: Injury patterns and treatment. *Arthroscopy* 1990;6:125–132.
8. Palmer AK, Werner FW. The triangular fibrocartilage complex of the wrist—anatomy and function. *J Hand Surg* 1981;6:153–162.
9. Palmer AK, Whipple TL, Poehling GG. Arthroscopy of the distal radioulnar joint. In: McGinty JB, Caspari RW, Jackson RW, Poehling GG, eds. *Operative Arthroscopy.* New York: Raven Press, 1991, pp. 659–662.
10. Poehling GG, Siegel DB, Koman LA, Chabon SJ. Arthroscopy of the wrist and elbow. In: Green DB, ed. *Operative Hand Surgery.* 3rd Ed. New York: Churchill Livingstone, 1993, pp. 189–214.
11. Roth JH, Haddad RG. Radiocarpal arthroscopy and arthrography in the diagnosis of ulnar wrist pain. *Arthroscopy* 1986;2:234–243.

Arthroscopy of the Distal Radioulnar Joint

Andrew K. Palmer, M.D., *Terry L. Whipple*, M.D., *and Gary G. Poehling*, M.D.

Arthroscopic examination of the distal radioulnar joint (DRUJ) is difficult. The radioulnar articulation is tight and cannot be separated or distracted. The usual distraction of the carpus for arthroscopic examination of the radiocarpal or midcarpal spaces tightens the radiocarpal capsule and further compresses the radioulnar articulation, much as a Chinese finger trap tightens circumferentially when it is pulled. Pronation and supination of the forearm pull tight either the dorsal or the volar portions of the distal radioulnar joint capsule, respectively, further compressing the joint as well. Thus, there is little

means of increasing the space in the DRUJ for insertion or manipulation of instruments.

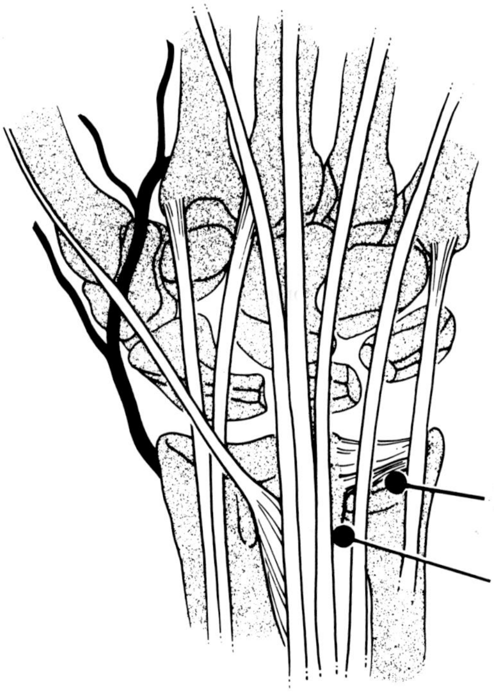

Still, there are small pockets of space in the DRUJ that can be entered when the joint capsule is distended. In supination, the ulna head shifts volarly in the sigmoid notch of the radius, and the dorsal capsule is simultaneously relaxed (2,4). This position provides an accessible space dorsally (portal DRUJ-2) for the introduction of arthroscopic instruments (Fig. 1).

There is also a space between the distal end of the ulna and the proximal surface of the central triangular fibrocartilage articular disc (TFC) of the triangular fibrocartilage complex (TFCC). The TFC is suspended from the sigmoid notch of the radius and the ulnar side of the carpus, and it sweeps over the end of the ulna in pronation and supination. The radius is relatively longer at the wrist compared with the ulna in supination, and supination "lifts" the radial side of the TFC away from the ulnar head (2,4). Thus, this narrow space (portal DRUJ-1) may be accessible in supination, especially in cases of relatively negative ulnar variance.

INDICATIONS

Arthroscopy of the distal radioulnar joint may be indicated for diagnostic or treatment purposes.

Because indirect imaging procedures are often inadequate or inconclusive for small soft tissue lesions of the DRUJ (6), examination by direct visualization may be advantageous. However, symptoms in the DRUJ that are aggravated by pronation, supination, or joint compression, and that can be functionally limiting, still may not justify the morbidity associated with arthrotomy, which disrupts the dorsal DRUJ capsular ligaments that contribute to rotational stability in pronation. Arthroscopic examination, when feasible, allows visualization

FIG. 1. Portals of the distal radioulnar joint (DRUJ).

DRUJ 1
DRUJ 2

of the articular cartilage of the ulnar head and the sigmoid notch, the proximal surface of the TFCC, the ulnar origin of the volar ulnocarpal ligaments (occasionally), and the synovial lining of the joint.

Articular lesions of the DRUJ are not commonly related to attrition or degeneration alone. When the articular surface of this joint shows signs or symptoms of arthrosis with deterioration of hyaline cartilage and marginal spur formation, usually there has been some antecedent history of crushing trauma, fracture, or distal radioulnar joint instability. Although chronic repeated pronation and supination may cause symptoms in the extensor carpi ulnaris and its retinaculum, they rarely cause deterioration of the joint.

Fractures of the distal radius that are incompletely reduced—especially Colles' and die-punch fractures—can alter the articular harmony of the ulna with the sigmoid notch of the radius. In such circumstances, degenerative arthritis of the DRUJ may result (3,5). Similarly, abnormal anterior–posterior translation of the head of the ulna, as encountered in DRUJ instability, can produce excessive wear. Which structures control DRUJ stability is not completely clear. Arthroscopy has permitted well-controlled isolated and combined cutting studies, which have demonstrated that the TFC plays little, if any, role as a DRUJ stabilizer (7). Cutting even the volar and dorsal edges of the TFCC did not cause instability with stressed pronation and supination. Nevertheless, instability of the DRUJ can lead to degenerative articular changes.

When there is strong clinical suspicion of intraarticular lesions in the DRUJ that may require surgical instrumentation, arthroscopy permits confirmation of the diagnosis before resorting to arthrotomy, or may even allow the treatment of certain problems percutaneously, thereby obviating the need for arthrotomy. When that possibility seems likely, arthroscopy may be a more appropriate diagnostic procedure than magnetic resonance imaging or arthrography, because of the opportunity to provide definitive treatment at the same time.

Typically, spur formation occurs on the dorsoulnar edge of the radial epiphysis. The sigmoid notch may deepen slightly with osteophyte formation, but this is not a common feature. Loose bodies may be found in the DRUJ. These occur also in the acute stages of comminuted distal radius fractures.

Chondromalacia of the head of the ulna is common (4). It probably reflects excessive compression against the carpus, but is not always symptomatic and need not necessarily be treated. When it is symptomatic, however, and when encountered in the presence of a TFC tear and ulnocarpal impaction syndrome, a leveling procedure can be performed.

Nontraumatic osteochondral defects in the DRUJ are usually associated with rheumatoid arthritis. The classic penciling of the distal ulna results from synovial hypertrophy and pannus infiltration of the bone. Obviously, removal of this pannus, whether by chemical or surgical means, is desirable. In contrast, once the ulnar head becomes soft from synovial invasion and subcondylar fractures occur in the DRUJ, arthroscopic treatment is of limited value. Although joint debridement and lavage may provide temporary pain relief, efforts should be directed primarily toward control of the synovial hypertrophy and pannus formation and toward preservation of motion.

TECHNIQUE

The forearm must be held in supination to relax the dorsal capsule, to move the ulna head volarly, and to lift the central articular disc distally from the head of the ulna. Distal traction should be reduced to 1–2 pounds, just enough to suspend the forearm vertically but not to compress the radioulnar articulation further. The DRUJ is initially distended with fluid from a hypodermic needle inserted at the DRUJ-2 portal site. However, if there is a large defect in the TFCC, fluid inflow through the radiocarpal space will distend the joint.

Through the DRUJ-1 portal, the arthroscope sheath and trocar are inserted with a twisting motion to enter between the head of the ulna and the TFCC. Care must be taken to avoid penetration of the TFC. While inflow is maintained on the sheath of the arthroscope, the arthroscope can be rotated or panned to show the origin of the volar ulnocarpal ligament ulnarly and the distal edge of the sigmoid notch radially, but the wrist should not be pronated. Rotating the lens of the arthroscope to look distally will show the proximal surface of the central disc.

For the DRUJ-2 portal to be entered, the forearm is supinated and the arthroscope sheath and trocar are inserted, aiming toward the sigmoid notch distally. It is difficult to avoid introduction of air into the joint as the arthroscope sheath is aimed upward; however, if pressure is maintained on the inflow line while the trocar is being withdrawn slowly from the sheath, the problem will be minimal. The arthroscope can be moved to follow the neck of the ulna proximally to the axilla of the joint capsule, and then distally to show the dorsal aspect of the sigmoid notch. Gentle pronation will parade the circumference of the ulnar head before the scope.

Indirect access to the DRUJ is possible in cases where central perforations exist in the TFC. The arthroscope can be advanced across the radiocarpal joint and through the TFC defect to show the sigmoid notch from the 6R portal, or to show the distal end of the ulna from the 3–4

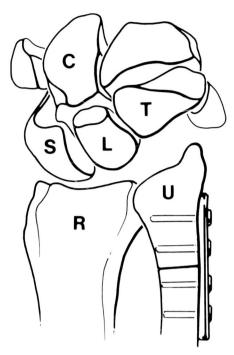

FIG. 2. Extraarticular shortening. C, capitate; L, lunate; R, radius; S, scaphoid; T, triquetrum; U, ulna. (From Palmer, ref. 2.)

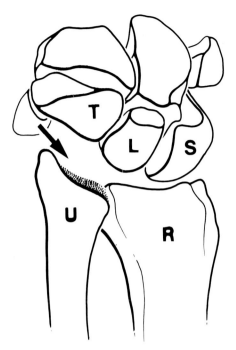

FIG. 3. Intraarticular wafer procedure. For abbreviations, see legend to Fig. 2. (From Palmer, ref. 2.)

portal. TFC defects are frequently associated with DRUJ disease. It may be necessary to enlarge the central defect in the TFC somewhat to gain sufficient arthroscopic visualization of the articular surface of the ulnar head. This apparently produces no ill effect.

Whether the arthroscope is introduced directly into the DRUJ or indirectly through a TFC defect, the forearm must be pronated and supinated to provide a circumferential view of the ulnar head. In either approach, the arthroscope should be held stationary relative to the radius and is rotated about the ulna circumferentially.

Osteophytes on the neck of the ulna or at the edge of the sigmoid notch can be seen only with the direct approach. In large wrists, a second portal can be established dorsally just proximal or distal to the DRUJ-2 portal to permit introduction of a powered bur or a $\frac{1}{8}$-inch chisel to resect the osteophytes.

If loose bodies are present in the DRUJ, they will usually "sink" to the axilla of the joint, being heavier than the irrigation fluid. Use of a second portal dorsally will usually admit a small grasping forceps to remove them.

As noted, in cases of ulnocarpal abutment in which the TFC has been perforated, a leveling procedure to shorten the distal end of the ulna can be performed. This may be accomplished extraarticularly by an ulnar shortening (Fig. 2) or intraarticularly by either an arthrotomy

or by arthroscopy (1,7) (Fig. 3). The defect in the TFC is enlarged to allow good visualization from the radiocarpal space. A $\frac{3}{16}$-inch chisel is then introduced through the dorsal capsule of the DRUJ or through an accessory radiocarpal portal, and a wafer of ulnar head approximately $\frac{1}{8}$-inch thick is resected while viewing through the TFC defect. Fragments are reduced piecemeal. Alternatively, a bur can be used to resect the distal aspect of the ulna head (Fig. 4). This is best accomplished by placing the arthroscope directly into the DRUJ and inserting the bur through the TFC defect. Every effort should be made not to leave debris in either the DRUJ or the radiocarpal joint space.

One of the most common posttraumatic bony defects on the ulnar side of the wrist—nonunion of the ulnar styloid—is not currently being treated under arthroscopic control. However, with greater experience, it may be possible to address this lesion in the future.

SUMMARY

The DRUJ is one of the least visible spaces in the wrist, and the most difficult space to access arthroscopically, yet arthroscopic examination of this joint, when possible, complements other diagnostic means and provides advantageous surgical approaches to some lesions.

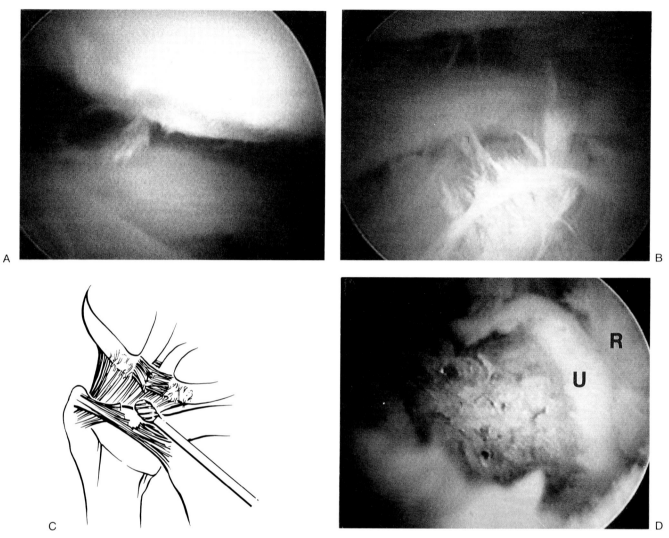

FIG. 4. Arthroscopic pre- and postulnar shortening. Defect in TFC with abrader taking off top of ulna (U). R, radius.

REFERENCES

1. Buterbaugh GA, Palmer AK. Fractures and dislocations of the distal radioulnar joint. *Hand Clin* 1988;4:361–375.
2. Ekenstam F. The distal radioulnar joint—an anatomical, experimental, and clinical study. *Acta Univ Abstr Uppsala,* Dissertation from the Faculty of Medicine 1984;505:1–55.
3. Palmer AK, Werner FW. Biomechanics of the distal radioulnar joint. *Clin Orthop* 1984;187:26–35.
4. Palmer AK. Triangular fibrocartilage afflictions: Injury patterns and treatment. *Arthroscopy* 1990;2:125–132.
5. Palmer AK. Fractures of the distal radius. In: Green DP, ed. *Operative Hand Surgery.* 2nd Ed. New York: Churchill Livingstone, 1988, vol. 2, pp. 991–1026.
6. Roth JH, Haddad RG. Radiocarpal arthroscopy and arthrography in the diagnosis of ulnar wrist pain. *Arthroscopy* 1986;2:234–243.
7. Whipple TL, Martin D, Yates C. The role of the triangular fibrocartilage in the stabilization of the DRUJ. AAOS Academy Meeting, February 1990, New Orleans.

Fractures of the Distal Forearm

L. Andrew Koman, M.D., and Gary G. Poehling, M.D.

The management of fractures of the distal radius and ulna has changed dramatically over the last two decades (1–5,7,11,15,17,24,26,28,30). Historically, treatment of these common injuries was directed primarily to the preservation of hand and finger function, with much less attention being paid to skeletal alignment of the radius and ulna. This basic tenet—"that the limb will at some remote period again enjoy perfect freedom in all its motions, [and] be completely exempt from pain regardless of deformity" (6)—is no longer considered appropriate. All too frequently, the sequelae of distal forearm fractures are chronic wrist pain, posttraumatic arthritis, or both (8,23,25,29,31,32). The purpose of this chapter is to describe the osseous and nonosseous intraarticular injuries associated with distal forearm fractures and to delineate the role of wrist arthroscopy in optimizing their management.

ASSESSMENT OF DISTAL FOREARM INJURY BY PLAIN ROENTGENOGRAPHY

Classification/Mechanism of Injury

Current classifications of distal forearm fractures relate to the initial displacement of the fragment(s) (Table 1), extraarticular vs. intraarticular involvement, and the presence or absence of a fracture of the distal ulna (10,13,14,18,20–22,30). These classifications are based on roentgenographic criteria and do not take into account quantitative osseous comminution or factors not visible on plain roentgenograms, such as articular cartilage damage, joint surface malalignment, associated intraarticular ligament disruption, and periarticular ligamentous damage. Although the associated scapholunate

ligament damage seen in some radial styloid fractures is well described, only recently has the extent of periarticular and structural damage to nonossified structures been delineated (16,19).

Nonetheless, Melone's classification is most appropriate when arthroscopic treatment of distal radial fractures is being considered. Melone classifies intraarticular fractures into four types, based on the relationships of the proximal radius, radial styloid, posterior medial radius, and anterior medial radius (20,21).

Type I (Fig. 1A) is an anatomic intraarticular fracture or a fracture that is stable after anatomic reduction. Type II (Fig. 1B) is an unstable fracture and it may present with a dorsally displaced posterior medial fragment or with a palmarly displaced anterior medial fragment. Type III (Fig. 1C)—the so-called spike fracture—is similar to type II, but includes a concomitant nerve or tendon injury secondary to the displacement of the proximal radius. Type IV (Fig. 1D)—the "split fracture"—is characterized by a wide separation of the anterior and posterior medial fragments.

TABLE 1. *Wrist fractures*

Type of fracture	Displacement	Mechanism
Colles	Dorsal radial	Fall on outstretched hand
Barton	Dorsal rim	Forced dorsiflexion and pronation of distal forearm on fixed wrist
Smith	Volar radial	Dorsiflexion and pronation on palmar flexion
	Radiocarpal dislocation	Pronation of forearm on fixed hand
Hutchinson	Radial styloid	Avulsion

Type I

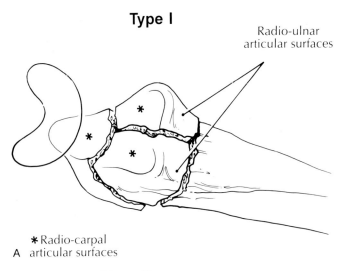

Radio-ulnar
articular surfaces

*Radio-carpal
A articular surfaces

Type II

Posterior Displacement

Anterior Displacement

B

Type III

Type IV

Dorsal medial
rotation

Nerve or tendon

Palmar medial
rotation

C

Spike fragment

D

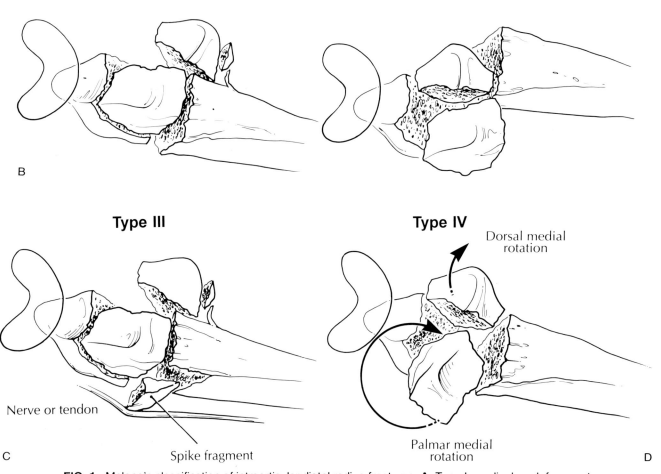

FIG. 1. Melone's classification of intraarticular distal radius fractures. **A:** Type I nondisplaced, four-part fractures, which have four fragments: dorsal and palmar medial fragment, radial, styloid fragment, as well as the proximal radius. These are considered stable. **B:** Type II fractures are of two types: the dorsal posterior displacement, which is the classical die punch fracture, and the anterior displacement. **C:** Type III fractures are similar to type II fractures but have a spike impaling the carpal canal structures. **D:** Type IV fractures have displacement of both medial fragments.

Incidence of Intraarticular Lesions

The extent of significant intraarticular injuries associated with extraarticular wrist fractures is difficult to assess with plain roentgenograms, which may account for many of the unexpected "bad results" so frequently observed (18). The incidence of intraarticular associated injuries see by arthroscopic assessment suggests that displaced fractures of the radius (Frykman III–VIII) have a 40% to 80% incidence of intraosseous ligament disruptions and/or triangular fibrocartilaginous complex tears (Table 2) (16,19). In addition, full-thickness and partial-thickness articular cartilage lesions, osseous cartilaginous chip fractures, loose bodies, unrecognized joint impactions, and articular malalignments may not be appreciated on plain roentgenograms and if not treated may result in later pain and/or functional compromise.

Prediction of Outcome

The results of less than optimal anatomic restoration of distal radioulnar architecture are well established (9). Failure to achieve appropriate length and proper inclination of articular joint surfaces may result in decreased wrist motion, loss of forearm rotation, intercarpal pain, and weakness secondary to intercarpal and distal radioulnar imbalances. Unrecognized and/or unrepaired ligamentous damage, cartilaginous disruption, or small loose osseous fragments may contribute additional damage and result in pain and posttraumatic arthritis (25,27,29,32).

Factors determining long-term outcome in fractures of the distal forearm include (a) skeletal alignment, (b) joint congruity, and (c) extent of ligamentous integrity (Table 3). Of these, only skeletal alignment can be assessed adequately by plain roentgenograms, the current standard postreduction assessment. Evaluation of patients with chronic wrist pain following trauma suggests that damage to the cartilage, including small osseous cartilaginous chips, cartilaginous loose bodies, impaction of the distal radius, or carpal or radial cartilage lesions, is

TABLE 2. *Arthroscopic assessment of intraarticular damage associated with distal radius fractures (Frykman III → VIII)*

Damage	Hanker	Kolkin
Scapholunate:		
Complete	6/30 (20%)	5/14 (36%)
Incomplete	7/30 (24%)	
Radioscapholunate:		
Complete	2/30 (6%)	
Incomplete	25/30 (83%)	
Triangular fibrocartilage tears	18/30 (60%)	
Ulnolunate	7/30 (24%)	
Lunotriquetral	0 (0)	2/14 (7%)
Dorsal capsular tear	22/30 (74%)	
Loose body	10/30 (35%)	

TABLE 3. *Factors related to outcome in distal forearm fractures*

Anatomic alignment
Cartilage damage
Ligamentous integrity
  Intracarpal
  Capsular
Triangular fibrocartilage intact
Stable distal radioulnar joint

difficult to assess by conventional plain roentgenography and accounts for a high incidence of long-term problems. In the case of *intraarticular fractures,* it also is difficult to determine definitive articular cartilage alignment or the presence or absence of capsular or intercapsular ligamentous damage, including disruption of the triangular fibrocartilage or distal radioulnar joint subluxation/dislocation. Magnetic resonance (MR) imaging and tomographic techniques alone or in combination provide some additional information. However, the definitive recognition of associated intraarticular or periarticular ligament damage is possible only by direct evaluation, and for that arthroscopy provides superior accuracy with less morbidity than arthrotomy.

In the current evaluation of *extraarticular injuries,* noninvasive modalities (including next-generation MR imaging) are not capable of providing definitive information, and data are insufficient to justify surgical or arthroscopic exploration of nondisplaced extraarticular fractures. As noninvasive modalities improve, and if appropriate outcome studies suggest significant unappreciated and thus nontreated lesions associated with extraarticular fractures, then wrist arthroscopy not only will be appropriate for diagnosis but may also become the standard of care.

CURRENT ARTHROSCOPIC PROCEDURES

Intraarticular Fractures

Arthroscopic treatment may not be appropriate for all distal radial fractures (12). The role of arthroscopy in nondisplaced or stable intraarticular fractures (i.e., Melone type I) has not yet been established, although the above data suggest its potential efficacy in any intraarticular injury in order (a) to document anatomic reconstruction of articular surfaces, (b) to determine the extent of ligamentous damage, and (c) to ensure that fracture debris is not left within the joint. However, the current standard of care does not demand arthroscopic or sophisticated noninvasive evaluation of stable reduced intraarticular fractures confirmed by plain roentgenography and treated by cast immobilization. If persistent mechanical symptoms occur after mobilization, arthroscopy may be considered during the follow-up period.

Displaced posterior medial radial fractures with dorsal

displacement (Melone's type II) (Fig. 1B) may be managed by arthroscopic intervention. Once the displaced "die punch" fracture is visualized directly, the joint can be debrided and the disimpaction and reduction confirmed. This bone should be stabilized and ligamentous injury recognized and treated. Provisional reduction is first achieved by manipulation and a distraction device (see Fig. 2). The joint is visualized arthroscopically and reduced and stabilized using an external fixator (see Fig. 3) with K-wires added as necessary, or open reduction (see Fig. 5). The use of a bone graft is optional.

Fractures of the anterior medial radial complex displaced palmarly (Melone's type II) (Fig. 1B) are difficult to treat arthroscopically, and often open reduction with a rigid palmar buttress plate is necessary to align and adequately stabilize the fracture fragments. Arthrotomy may be avoided by employing the arthroscope to debride the joint and identify and/or treat any associated ligamentous injuries of the wrist.

The volarly displaced "spike" fracture (Melone's type III) (Fig. 1C) may be treated identically to the dorsal type II fracture after open exploration of the flexor compartment and management of any nerve or tendon injuries.

A fracture splitting the medial fragments of the distal radius (Melone's type IV) generally requires open reduction and internal fixation for a reassembling of the fragments. Both a palmar and a dorsal approach may be

needed. Frequently, bone grafts are needed to fill large defects. Arthroscopy may be used in place of arthrotomy, thus decreasing the amount of dissection and additional ligamentous damage, yet allowing joint debridement, assessment of joint congruity following reduction, and evaluation of associated injuries.

Extravasation of fluid into an acutely injured extremity is of practical concern during arthroscopic intervention in the wrist and may be decreased by (a) delaying the procedure for 24–96 hr, (b) wrapping the proximal extremity during the procedure, (c) employing a pressure control pump for distension, and (d) ensuring careful postarthroscopic management. Arthroscopic evaluation in the presence of acute median nerve compression should be performed with caution unless simultaneous nerve decompression is planned.

The 3–4, 6R, and 4–5 portals provide optimal wrist access for the arthroscope and accessory instruments. In most cases, outflow and pressure monitoring are established through the 6R portal and the arthroscope is inserted through the 3–4 portal. If skeletal alignment is to be established by closed reduction and maintained by application of an external fixator, pins should be placed and provisional fixation and/or traction (Fig. 2) should be obtained before the arthroscopic evaluation (Figs. 3 and 4). If open reduction with internal fixation is chosen, then the arthroscopic evaluation may proceed using trac-

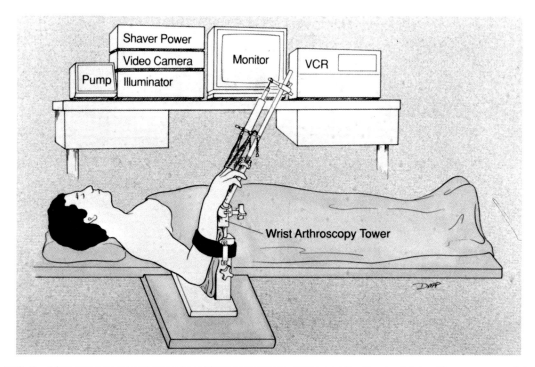

FIG. 2. After provisional reduction is achieved by manipulation and fixation is obtained by an appropriate external device (traction tower demonstrated), the arthroscope is introduced and the radiocarpal and midcarpal joints are evaluated for ligamentous damage, loose bodies, and joint reduction. Definitive fixation by pins, external fixation, internal fixation, or plaster immobilization is then used.

tion with fingertraps, using the standard portals, and introducing the arthroscope under direct vision (Fig. 5). Once the extent of intraarticular damage has been assessed, the treatment plan can be formulated to correct or protect associated soft tissue injuries and to effect definitive reduction with internal and external fixation.

Authors' Preferred Technique

We prefer to postpone arthroscopy of the fractured distal forearm 24 to 96 hours when bleeding has stopped and swelling is decreasing. Once the patient is in the operating room, appropriate regional or general anesthesia is established and the hand and forearm are exsanguinated. The tourniquet is inflated, traction is applied, and a preliminary reduction is obtained (Fig. 2). Inflow and outflow portals are established. A small-joint arthroscope is inserted through the 3–4 portal, and hand or power instruments are inserted through the 4–5 or 6R portal. The joint is irrigated, and clotted blood, fibrin, and joint debris are removed with a small shaver, grasping forceps, etc. The radiocarpal and midcarpal joints are

then evaluated and the extent of osseous and nonosseous injury is assessed. The extent of joint incongruity is noted (Fig. 6) and the steps of the reduction are planned. Careful evaluation of all capsular and ligamentous structures is important, and the intercarpal ligaments and triangular fibrocartilage complex are probed for partial tears or injury (Fig. 7). At this point, it is important to consider contingency approaches (a) to manage the soft tissue/ligamentous injury (or injuries); (b) to obtain provisional skeletal reduction; and (c) to accomplish rigid final bony stabilization. Arthroscopic-assisted reduction of joint surfaces (Fig. 8) and repair or removal of damaged soft ligamentous tissue is then achieved systematically.

After reduction, intraarticular fractures are stabilized with external fixation (Fig. 3). Blood, loose bodies, and debris are removed from the joint and the congruity of the articular surface(s) is reconfirmed. Additional percutaneous pins may be necessary to stabilize a fragment. The adequacy of treatment to injured soft tissues is assessed. Postoperatively the patient mobilizes as rapidly as the injuries will allow. External fixation is removed in 4–8 weeks.

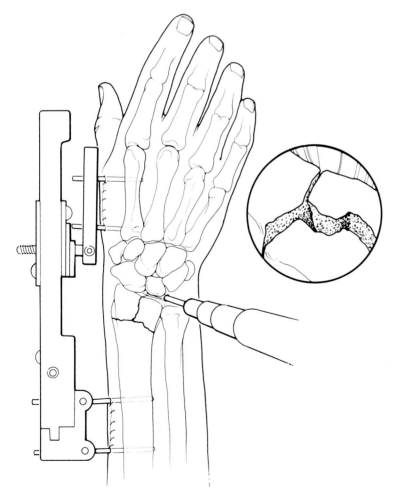

FIG. 3. Arthroscopic evaluation may be performed after definitive fixation to confirm reduction. Residual fracture displacement (**inset**) can be managed without removal of traction.

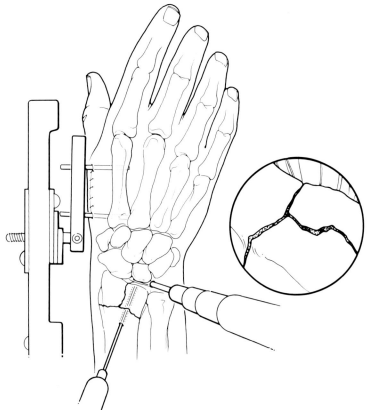

FIG. 4. With fixation in place, a percutaneous incision is used to drill a 5-mm cortical window in the radius in line with the depressed joint fragment. A blunt probe is then used to elevate the fragment until it is anatomically reduced. A subcortical transfixion pin may be used to secure the fragment.

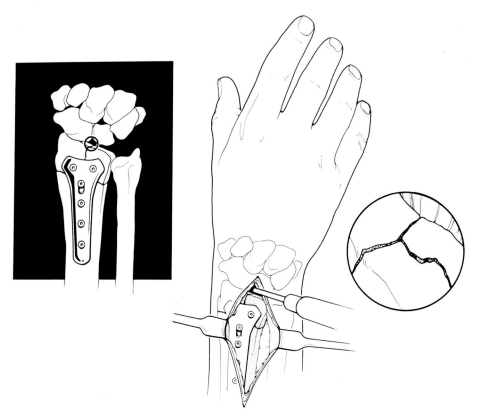

FIG. 5. If open reduction is employed, skeletal fixation is achieved and the arthroscope is inserted through the joint capsule without need for an extensive arthrotomy.

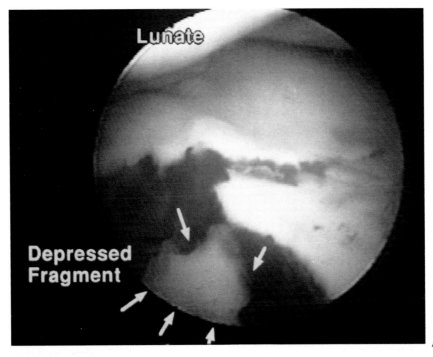

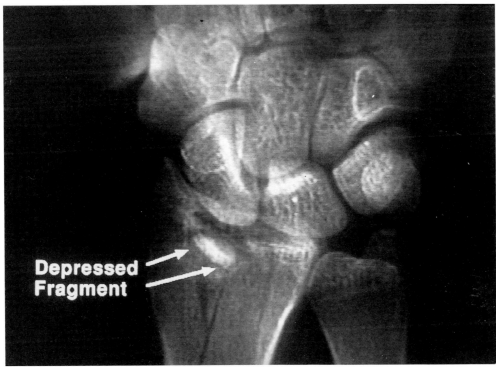

FIG. 6. Distal radius fracture before reduction (**A and B**).

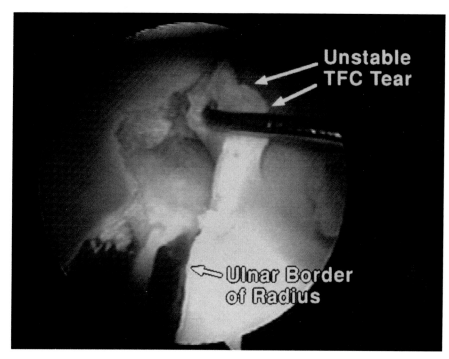

FIG. 7. Probe in triangular fibrocartilage tear associated with intraarticular fracture in Fig. 6.

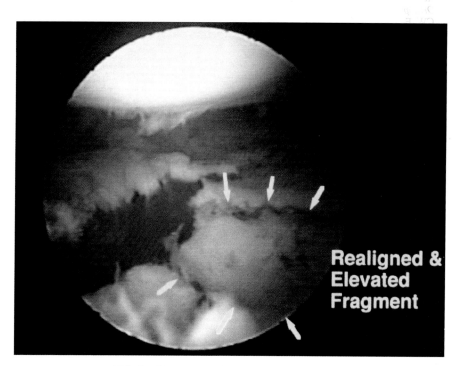

FIG. 8. Distal radius fracture after reduction.

REFERENCES

1. American Association of Orthopedic Surgeons. *Orthopedic Knowledge Update 3. Home Study Syllabus.* AAOS, 1990, p. 353.
2. Bassett RL. Displaced intraarticular fractures of the distal radius. *Clin Orthop* 1987;214:148–152.
3. Bradway JK, Amadio PC, Cooney WP. Open reduction and internal fixation of displaced, comminuted intraarticular fractures of the distal end of the radius. *J Bone Joint Surg* 1989;71A:839–847.
4. Chapman DR, Bennett JB, Bryan WJ, Tullos HS. Complications of distal radial fractures: Pins and plaster treatment. *J Hand Surg* 1982;7:509–512.
5. Cole JM, Obletz BE. Comminuted fractures of the distal end of the radius treated by skeletal transfixion in plaster cast. An end-result study of thirty-three cases. *J Bone Joint Surg* 1966;48A:931–945.
6. Colles A. On the fracture of the carpal extremity of the radius. *Edinb Med Surg J* 1814;10:182–186.
7. Cooney WP. External fixation of distal radius fractures. *Clin Orthop* 1983;180:44–49.
8. Cooney WP III, Dobyns JH, Linscheid RL. Complications of Colles' fractures. *J Bone Joint Surg* 1980;62A:613–619.
9. Cooney WP III, Linscheid RL, Dobyns JH. External pin fixation for unstable Colles' fractures. *J Bone Joint Surg* 1979;61A:840–845.
10. De Oliveira JC. Barton's fractures. *J Bone Joint Surg* 1973;55A:586–594.
11. Dobyns JH, Linscheid RL. Fractures and dislocations of the wrist. In: Rockwood CA Jr, Green DP, eds. *Fractures in Adults.* 2nd Ed. Philadelphia: JB Lippincott, 1984, pp. 411–509.
12. Easterling KJ, Wolfe SW. Wrist arthroscopy: An overview. *Contemp Orthop* 1992;24:21–30.
13. Frykman G. Fracture of the distal radius including sequelae—shoulder-hand-finger syndrome, disturbance of the distal radioulnar joint and impairment of nerve function. A clinical and experimental study. *Acta Orthop Scand Suppl* 1967;108:3–153.
14. Gartland JJ Jr., Werley CW. Evaluation of healed Colles' fractures. *J Bone Joint Surg* 1951;33A:895–907.
15. Green DP. Pins and plaster treatment of comminuted fractures of the distal end of the radius. *J Bone Joint Surg* 1975;57A:304–310.
16. Hanker GJ. Arthroscopic evaluation of intra-articular distal radius fractures. Presented at 46th Annual Meeting of the American Society for Surgery of the Hand, October 2–5, 1991.
17. Hubbard LF. Fractures of the hand and wrist. In: Evarts CMcC, ed. *Surgery of the Musculoskeletal System.* 2nd Ed. New York: Churchill Livingstone, 1990, pp. 349–383.
18. Knirk JL, Jupiter JB. Intra-articular fractures of the distal end of the radius in young adults. *J Bone Joint Surg* 1986;68A:647–659.
19. Kolkin J. The use of arthroscopy and percutaneous pin fixation for intra-articular fractures of the distal radius in young adults. Presented at the Bowman Gray 10th Annual Alumni Meeting, Winston-Salem, NC, October 1991.
20. Melone CP Jr. Articular fractures of the distal radius. *Orthop Clin North Am* 1984;15:217–236.
21. Melone CP Jr. Open treatment for displaced articular fractures of the distal radius. *Clin Orthop* 1986;202:103–111.
22. Older TM, Stabler EV, Cassebaum WH. Colles' fracture: Evaluation and selection of therapy. *J Trauma* 1965;5:469–476.
23. Posner MA, Ambrose L. Malunited Colles' fractures: Correction with a biplanar closing wedge osteotomy. *J Hand Surg* 1991;16A:1017–1026.
24. Sarmiento A, Pratt GW, Berry NC, Sinclair WF. Colles' fractures. Functional bracing in supination. *J Bone Joint Surg* 1975;57A:311–317.
25. Scheck M. Long-term follow-up of treatment of comminuted fractures of the distal end of the radius by transfixation with Kirschner wires and cast. *J Bone Joint Surg* 1962;44A:337–351.
26. Seitz WH Jr., Froimson AI, Leb R, Shapiro JD. Augmented external fixation of unstable distal radius fractures. *J Hand Surg* 1991;16A:1010–1016.
27. Short WH, Palmer AK, Werner FW, Murphy DJ. A biomechanical study of distal radial fractures. *J Hand Surg* 1987;12A:529–534.
28. Stein AH Jr, Katz SF. Stabilization of comminuted fractures of the distal inch of the radius: Percutaneous pinning. *Clin Orthop* 1975;108:174–181.
29. Taleisnik J, Watson HK. Midcarpal instability caused by malunited fractures of the distal radius. *J Hand Surg* 1984;9A:350–357.
30. Thomas FB. Reduction of Smith's fracture. *J Bone Joint Surg* 1957;39B:463–470.
31. Villar RN, Marsh D, Rushton N, Greatorex RA. Three years after Colles' fracture. A prospective review. *J Bone Joint Surg* 1987;69B:635–638.
32. Weber SC, Szabo RM. Severely comminuted distal radial fracture as an unsolved problem. Complications associated with external fixation and pins and plaster techniques. *J Hand Surg* 1986;11A:157–165.

Articular Cartilage Lesions of the Wrist

Gary G. Poehling, M.D., *and James H. Roth,* M.D.

Articular cartilage lesions in the wrist joint were rarely diagnosed before the advent of arthroscopy. A vast array of these lesions have now been identified arthroscopically. Articular (hyaline) cartilage is a type of connective tissue that bears weight and allows smooth gliding motions of the joint surface. The biomechanical properties of articular cartilage that enable it to perform these functions depend in part on its macromolecular organization and chemical composition.

Articular cartilage consists primarily of water and an extracellular ground substance composed of collagen and proteoglycans. Histologically, the only living components of articular cartilage, the chondrocytes, reside in the extracellular matrix.

BIOCHEMICAL ANATOMY

Articular cartilage contains type 2 collagen. Each molecule of type 2 collagen consists of alpha I (type 2) polypeptide chains that are coiled in a rigid triple helix (Fig.

1). Proteoglycans form the other structural component of the extracellular matrix of hyaline cartilage. These macromolecules consist of a core protein structure along which some 100 chondroitin sulfate chains and 30 to 60 keratin sulfate chains are arranged like the bristles of a brush (Fig. 2). Water molecules are attracted to the chains, which can then occupy solution volumes 30 to 50 times their dry volume. These chains then aggregate along a central filament of hyaluronic acid. They are cemented to the filament by a globular protein called a link protein (Fig. 3). The result is a very large structure that may immobilize the proteoglycans in the matrix and provide a network for the retention of large volumes of water.

It is felt that collagen restricts the flow of proteoglycans and preserves their colloidal properties. Therefore, collagen acts as an elastic element in sustaining compressive loads, while the reversibly compressible aggregates of proteoglycan provide the viscous qualities of cartilage (Fig. 4).

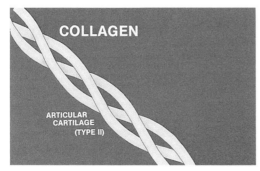

FIG. 1. Collagen, with its rigid triple helix, acts as the binding element in articular cartilage.

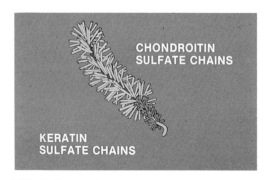

FIG. 2. Proteoglycans are macromolecules that consist of a core protein (*red*), chondroitin sulfate chain (*yellow*), and keratin sulfate chain (*green*).

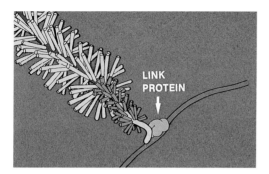

FIG. 3. The core protein with its chondroitin sulfate chains (*yellow*) and keratin sulfate chains (*green*), is cemented along a central filament of hyaluronic acid by a globular protein called a link protein (*blue*). This arrangement is repeated many times along the central filament, creating a huge hydrophilic structure.

HISTOLOGY

Articular cartilage is arranged in four zones. The first zone is a superficial layer in which small, flattened cells lie with their long axis parallel to the joint surface (Fig. 5). This layer acts as a shield to the underlying layers and is called the "lamina splendens." The second zone is a transitional layer in which the cells are more rounded. The third zone is a deep layer composed of plump columnar cells that lie in perpendicular rows between bundles of collagen fibers. The fourth zone is a calcified zone that is demarcated from the deep zone by a wavy line, the "tidemark," which stains blue with basic dye. This calcified zone rests on a thin layer of subchondral lamellar bone to which it is securely attached by the interdigitation and continuity of its fibrils with the fibrils of the underlying bone.

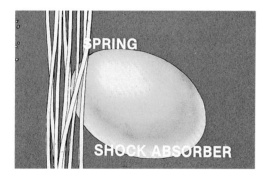

FIG. 4. There are two extracellular structural elements in articular cartilage. Their rigid collagen binds a compressible proteoglycans. Together they function as a substance that can absorb loads and maintain their shape.

FIG. 5. Four distinct zones of articular cartilage: *1*, superficial (lamina splendens); *2*, transitional zone; *3*, columnar zone; and *4*, calcified zone.

ARTICULAR DEGENERATION

Many theories have been proposed to explain the breakdown of articular cartilage, but a clear picture of the various stages involved can be drawn from the changes seen in osteoarthritis. The earliest identifiable defect in the articular cartilage is an increase in the water content of the matrix (1). This increase implies a failure of the elastic restraint of the collagen network, which would normally enable the proteoglycans to swell to a higher degree of hydration (Fig. 6) (9). In turn, this stimulates the chondrocytes to produce proteoglycans that are smaller and less tightly bound by the collagen and thus are more easily extracted from the cartilage (7). There is also a loss of orientation of the collagen fibers near the articular surface as individual fibers separate (1). Extrinsic factors can influence cartilage breakdown by direct proteolytic attack on the matrix or by stimulating the chondrocyte to release lysosomes that destroy the matrix (Fig. 7). Cartilage degeneration may be acceler-

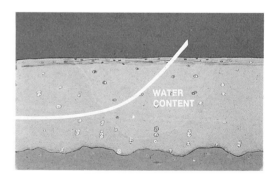

FIG. 6. The earliest changes in osteoarthritis demonstrate an increase in the water content of articular cartilage.

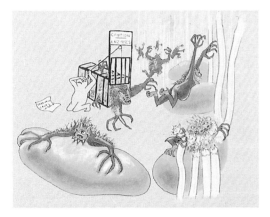

FIG. 7. Extrinsic factors such as excessive pressure or lack of any pressure may stimulate the chondrocyte to release lysosomes, which attack the collagen and the proteoglycans.

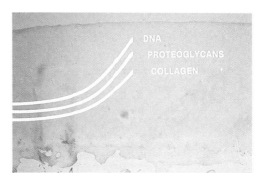

FIG. 8. The articular cartilage cells respond to the early degenerative changes by increased production of proteoglycans and collagen. While the production is up, the quality of the material produced is diminished.

ated by release of destructive enzymes from cells involved in the inflammatory response, exposure to immune complexes from which cartilage is normally isolated, and the formation of lymphokines in response to cell-mediated immune mechanisms (8).

These changes occur throughout the extent of the articular cartilage, before fibrillation or other morphologic change is evident, and while the proteoglycan content of the tissue is normal (5). During the early stages of degeneration the synthesis of both proteoglycans and collagen increases (Fig. 8). The synthesis of proteoglycan continues to rise to a point where the disease is far advanced, at which time the synthesis of proteoglycan decreases sharply and the chondrocytes fail (6).

Clinically, there are four grades of articular cartilage lesions (Fig. 9). Grade I corresponds to the increase in water content, with some laxity of the collagen meshwork. The articular cartilage appears normal but is soft to the touch. The lamina splendens remains intact.

In grade II, the lamina splendens erodes and early fibrillation and superficial disruption of the articular car-

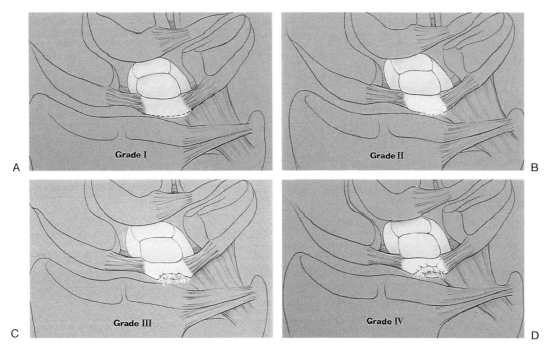

FIG. 9. A: Grade I lesion has an intact lamina splendens, is slightly swollen, and is soft to palpation. B: Grade II demonstrates erosion of the lamina splendens in early fibrillation. C: Grade III fissuring into the deeper layers of the articular cartilage is evident. D: Grade IV reveals exposed bone.

tilage occur. If degradation continues, fissures will form in the deep layers of the articular cartilage, causing separation and loss of biomechanical strength (grade III). Grade IV is represented by the erosion of all cartilaginous surfaces to the bone.

TREATMENT OF WRIST LESIONS

Degenerative Lesions

Antiinflammatory agents provide symptomatic relief and reduce the synovitis that is present. It is our impression that in the early stages of disease of the joints, salicylates, nonsteroidal antiinflammatories, and other substances that influence cartilage and its environment may be used to neutralize the causative factors (8,12,14). This may allow healing of the collagen and lamina splendens, thereby stabilizing the underlying chondrocytes. However, some authors believe that these drugs may contribute to degenerative changes in the articular cartilage and bone (2,3,10,11,13).

Even with the use of antiinflammatory agents, however, healing will fail if debris irritates the articular surface. At a given point, the degradative process becomes self-perpetuating due to mechanical irritation. Drug therapy seems to lose its effect at this point. All mechanical factors, including torn cartilage, loose bodies, malalignments, and instabilities, must be corrected promptly to prevent cartilage degradation. Treatment of degenerative articular cartilage lesions should begin by decreasing the forces across the softened articular cartilage (2). It is at this point that arthroscopy is useful. Arthroscopy can be used to wash out debris and the lysosomal enzymes that destroy the articular surface, thereby encouraging healing of the lamina splendens, tightening of the meshwork of the collagen (preventing the escape of proteoglycans), and stabilizing the chondrocytes and their surrounding matrix.

Traumatic Lesions

Traumatic lesions of articular cartilage are divided into three basic types; partial thickness, full thickness, and extension into subchondral bone. The treatment differs for each.

A scuff with the arthroscope removes just the upper levels of the articular surface in a partial-thickness lesion (Fig. 10). This disturbance seems to stimulate the underlying chondrocytes to increase their activity and to reform the four layers of articular cartilage. The irregular surface left by the defect does not appear to have any long-term deleterious effect on the joint.

Full-thickness lesions will not heal because the cartilaginous cells are absent. Also, when the collagen fibers

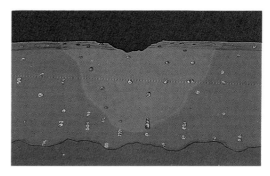

FIG. 10. Traumatic partial-thickness lesion of articular cartilage heals by reforming the four layers with a diminished volume.

that attach the articular cartilage to the subchondral bone are disrupted, that cartilage will never effectively reattach itself to bone but will remain as a loose fragment (Fig. 11). The fate of full-thickness lesions of articular cartilage depends on the strength of the edges of the lesions and the mechanical disruption within the joint. Therefore, it is important to remove any articular cartilage that has been detached from the bone, as well as any mechanical debris within the joint itself.

The treatment of exposed subchondral bone in severe articular cartilaginous degeneration is a subject of controversy (4,15). Abrasion chondroplasty initiates the production of fibrocartilage and has a moderate improvement rate with a low incidence of morbidity that many practitioners feel justifies the use of this procedure. Others feel that debridement or irrigation of the joint is logical, but the focus of attention should be on correcting the mechanical abnormalities that are causing the degeneration.

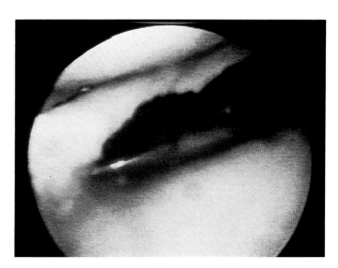

FIG. 11. A full-thickness articular cartilage lesion with separation from the lunate. Once the collagen fibers that bind articular cartilage to the bone are disrupted, that articular cartilage will remain loose.

Articular Cartilage Wrist Lesions

Lesions of the articular cartilage that extend into subchondral bone are most often the result of interarticular fractures. The removal of debris and the restoration of the joint surface are critical to successful treatment. Lesions with subchondral bone penetration will heal with a vascular proliferative response that results in fibrocartilage production.

CLINICAL REVIEW

A retrospective review of the experience of three institutions was undertaken from February 1984 to July 1987 to determine the frequency and location of articular cartilage lesions. The 73 patients included 41 women and 32 men, ranging in age from 13 to 71 years (average age 35 years). The dominant wrist was involved in 42% of the cases. All patients had experienced wrist pain for more than 3 months or had acute injuries with visible interarticular fractures or instabilities. All patients underwent standard clinical and radiographic evaluation.

Cartilage lesions were classified as primary if the source of symptoms was judged to be from the articular cartilage and secondary if the source of the articular cartilage lesion was other than articular cartilage, that is, due to ligament instability, triangular fibrocartilage (TFC) perforation, or avascular necrosis.

Arthroscopic examinations discovered 74 lesions in 73 wrists during this period. Fewer than one-third of these lesions were suspected prior to undergoing arthroscopy. A total of 82 lesions were identified. Of 40 primary lesions of articular cartilage, there were 18 TFC tears that were judged not to have caused the articular lesion nor to be the primary cause of symptoms. Radiocarpal defects were most commonly observed in the distal radius and the lunate. There were 34 wrists with secondary lesions. These lesions tended to be found in the midcarpal joint and involved the tip of the hamate, triquetrum, and lunate (Fig. 12).

Based on objective and subjective criteria, 71% of the patients had improvement. Those patients with primary lesions experienced 83% improvement, while those with secondary lesions had only a 55% incidence of improvement.

Complications included two temporary exacerbations of previous reflex sympathetic dystrophy and one extravasation of fluid, which resolved with elevation and compression.

Articular cartilage defects are difficult to diagnose without the use of arthroscopy. In an independent series, articular cartilage lesions were found to be associated with fractures, tears of the TFC, ligament instability, and 30% of the time to be isolated, for a total 64% incidence rate.

In summary, articular cartilage lesions are a common cause of wrist pain. Our data suggest that arthroscopic

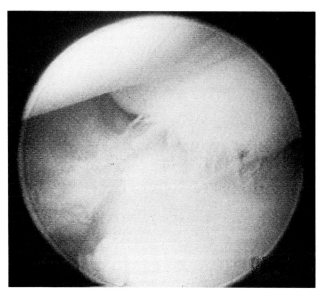

FIG. 12. Grade III lesion of the tip of the hamate, with common early degeneration in the wrist. It appears to be more common in patients who have a hamate facet of the lunate.

treatment of primary lesions by debridement is helpful in a high percentage of patients. It further suggests that debridement is of limited value in secondary lesions and that TFC perforations do not necessarily produce wrist pain. Wrist arthroscopy is accurate, has a low morbidity rate, provides a technique for timely intervention, and will give us a greater understanding of the development of interarticular problems within the wrist.

REFERENCES

1. Brandt KD. Pathogenesis of osteoarthritis. In: Kelley WN, Harris ED Jr, Ruddy S, Sledge CB, eds. *Textbook of Rheumatology.* Vol. 2. 2nd Ed. Philadelphia: WB Saunders, 1985, pp. 1417–1431.
2. Brandt KD. Management of osteoarthritis. In: Kelley WN, Harris ED Jr, Ruddy S, Sledge CB, eds. *Textbook of Rheumatology.* Vol. 2. 2nd Ed. Philadelphia: WB Saunders, 1985, pp. 1448–1458.
3. Brandt KD, Slowman-Kovacs S. Nonsteroidal antiinflammatory drugs in treatment of osteoarthritis. *Clin Orthop* 1986;213:84–91.
4. Johnson LL. Arthroscopic abrasion arthroplasty historical and pathological perspective: present status. *Arthroscopy* 1986;2:54–69.
5. Kempson GE, Muir H, Swanson SAV, Freeman MAR. Correlations between the compressive stiffness and chemical constituents of human articular cartilage. *Biochem Biophys Acta* 1970;215:70.
6. Mankin HJ. The response of articular cartilage to mechanical injury. *J Bone Joint Surg [Am]* 1982;64:460–466.
7. McDevitt CA, Billingham MEJ, Muir H. In vivo metabolism of proteoglycans in experimental osteoarthritis and normal canine articular cartilage and the intervertebral disc. *Semin Arthritis Rheum* 1981;11(Suppl 1):17–18.
8. Moskowitz RW. Which comes first: Inflammation or osteoarthritis? *J Rheumatol* 1983;Suppl 9:57–58.
9. Muir H. Proteoglycans: State of the art. *Semin Arthritis Rheum* 1981;11(Suppl 1):7–10.

10. Palmoski M, Brandt KD. Effects of some nonsteroidal antiinflammatory drugs on proteoglycan metabolism and organization in canine articular cartilage. *Arthritis Rheum* 1980;23:1010–1020.

11. Palmoski M, Brandt KD. In vivo effect of aspirin on canine osteoarthritic cartilage. *Arthritis Rheum* 1983;26:994–1001.

12. Poehling GG, White M. Partial-thickness defects of articular cartilage. *Field of View: Orthop/Arthrosc* 1983;2:1–5.

13. Ronningen H, Langeland N. Indomethacin treatment in osteoarthritis of the hip joint. *Acta Orthop Scand* 1979;50:169–174.

14. Simmons DP, Chrisman OD. Salicylate inhibition of cartilage degeneration. *Arthritis Rheum* 1965;8:960–969.

15. Sledge CB. Arthroscopic chondroabrasion: rational/irrational? Keynote address, American Academy of Orthopedic Surgeons Summer Institute, September 9, 1985, New York.

Inflammatory Arthritis of the Wrist

Donald C. Ferlic, M.D., *and William P. Cooney*, M.D.

Since 1985 there have been remarkable advancements in the art of joint arthroscopy and there has been significant progress within the field of arthroscopy of the wrist. Arthroscopy of the wrist has been useful primarily in the diagnosis and treatment of traumatic injuries. The role of arthroscopy in the evaluation of inflammatory synovitis of the wrist has been less clearly defined; little has been written about its use in this disorder, with only Chin (2,3) reporting on his use of it in cases of rheumatoid arthritis. He used arthroscopy for judging the intensity and extent of pathologic changes and not for synovectomies or other operative procedures.

DIFFERENTIAL DIAGNOSIS

There are over 100 types of arthritis and rheumatic disorders, with rheumatoid arthritis second only to degenerative joint disease in occurrence. Patterns of joint involvement are helpful in the diagnosis of arthritis. Clinically, the disease is polyarticular and symmetrical. Typically, the small joints of the hands and feet swell initially, but wrist disease is almost invariably noted (8). Active synovitis can be observed on the dorsum of the wrist as boggy, soft tissue swelling. Median nerve compression may develop due to volar tenosynovitis. Later in the disease process, immobility results from fibrous or bony ankylosis. Commonly, forearm rotation is painful or limited due to distal radioulnar joint involvement.

Systemic lupus erythematosus (SLE) can present with wrist and hand deformities similar to rheumatoid arthritis. Joint involvement is the most common manifestation of SLE (9). Joint pain or swelling may precede the onset of this multisystem disease by many years. Arthritis with objective evidence of painful motion, tenderness,

or effusion is present in 75% of SLE patients at the time of diagnosis. The joints most commonly involved are the proximal interphalangeal joints, knees, wrists, and metacarpophalangeal joints. Joint involvement is remarkably symmetrical (8). Generally, the deformities are passively correctable, but over time they can also become fixed (6). The articular cartilage is usually well preserved until late in the disease, with joint spaces roentgenographically normal. These joints sometimes have severe deformities seen clinically, but the radiographs (4) may be normal.

Scleroderma is one of the components of progressive systemic sclerosis. Hand involvement is almost universal with this condition, as 98% of the patients have Reynaud's phenomenon (8). Polyarthralgias and joint stiffness affecting both small and large peripheral joints are common. Many patients develop severe deformities of the fingers and wrists due to intense fibrosis of the synovium. Radiographs reveal subcutaneous calcinosis as well as absorption of the tufts of the terminal phalanges. Other areas of bone absorption include the distal portions of the radius and ulna as well as the ribs and mandible (8).

Psoriatic arthritis classically affects the distal interphalangeal joints but can affect any of the joints, including the wrists. The pattern of symmetrical polyarthritis is clinically indistinguishable from rheumatoid arthritis. Arthritis mutilans may be a component; except for this condition, psoriatic arthritis tends to cause less pain and disability than rheumatoid arthritis. Belsky et al. (1) found that patterns of hand and wrist involvement differed from those typically seen in rheumatoid disease. Their patients had multiple joint involvement in the hands, with joint destruction and stiffness as characteristic findings, rather than the typical instability seen in rheumatoid arthritis. Palmar subluxation of the carpus, common in the rheumatoid patient, was not found, but spontaneous wrist fusion was common.

Osteoarthritis is the most common joint disease. This condition can be divided into primary and secondary depending on the presence of some pre-existing condition. While primary osteoarthritis commonly involves the thumb basal joints and the digits with Heberden's and Bouchard's nodes in the distal and proximal interphalangeal joints, wrist joint involvement is uncommon. Secondary degenerative arthritis of the wrist is very common due to old trauma.

Gouty arthritis is caused by sodium urate crystals in the synovium as a result of chronic hyperuremia. In the majority of patients, recurrent bouts of acute joint inflammation constitute the first manifestation of the disease, but in 10% to 15% of the patients, it is preceded by nephrolithiasis (8). A family history is common. It is a disease of middle-aged and older men, but women can also be affected. The initial attacks are typically monarticular and most often affect the great toe or other foot joints, ankles, and knees. The acute episode can be confused with sepsis because of the swelling, redness, heat, and temperature. The patient may also have a low-grade fever and leukocytosis. Initially, the attacks are separated by long periods of time, but as the disease progresses, they become more frequent and affect fingers, wrists, and elbows. Primarily, the joints return to normal during the remissions, but later, permanent, chronic arthritis persists. Before effective control of hyperuremia was available, up to 60% of gout patients developed tophi. Medical treatment with uricouric agents is usually all that is necessary to control or shrink gouty tophi, but it may be necessary to debride and decompress tendons and nerves involved with gouty tenosynovitis in the wrist (7,10).

Pseudogout caused by a deposition of calcium pyrophosphate crystals is marked by inflammation in one or more joints lasting for several days or longer. These episodes are usually self-limited and are less painful than gout (8). This disease can be similar to rheumatoid arthritis, with multiple symmetrical joint involvement lasting for weeks or months. The wrists are the second most commonly affected joints after the knees. Metacarpophalangeal joints, hips, shoulders, elbows, and ankles follow in occurrence. Flexion deformities develop. Radiographs demonstrate crystal deposition in articular fibrocartilage of the wrist (Fig. 1).

Infectious disease arthritis includes bacteremic and fungal involvement, which can proceed rapidly to destruction of articular cartilage if not recognized early. Septic arthritis from fungal infections and atypical myobacterium can be particularly difficult to diagnose and usually requires tissue for culture to be successfully recognized.

Some of the other conditions that result in wrist deformities similar to rheumatoid arthritis are juvenile

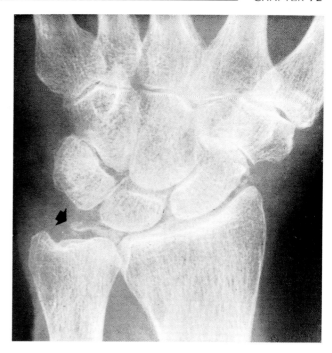

FIG. 1. Calcium pyrophosphate deposition in the fibrocartilage of the wrist.

rheumatoid arthritis, mixed connective tissue disease, ankylosing spondylitis, Reiter's syndrome, rheumatic fever with Jacoud's syndrome, sarcoidosis, and hemachromatosis (5).

INDICATIONS

The specific role of arthroscopy of the wrist in rheumatoid arthritis and other inflammatory conditions of the wrist involves two specific areas. The primary evidence has been the use of arthroscopy for the *diagnosis* of inflammatory conditions of the wrist. Specifically, arthroscopy can assist rheumatologists, physiatrists, and colleagues in infectious disease to obtain appropriate biopsy of the wrist synovium to confirm the diagnosis of rheumatoid arthritis, psoriatic arthritis, crystalline arthritis, and infectious monoarticular arthritis at a variety of stages of presentation. In several circumstances, patients have been referred specifically for arthroscopic examination because an accurate diagnosis of multisystem disease was not present. By using selected portals for wrist arthroscopy, one can separately biopsy the preradial styloid recess, the volar capsule beneath the radioscapholunate ligament, and the ulnar prestyloid recess and sacculus recessiformis. The articular cartilage can be inspected and probed for loss of substance, intraarticular cyst formation, and integrity of interosseous ligaments. Loose calcium or urate crystal deposits can be retrieved and then removed from a second arthroscopic portal. In addition, midcarpal biopsy can be performed through a separate portal and, with the combination of both radio-carpal and midcarpal arthroscopy, the condition of the articular cartilage can be carefully determined and cor-related with the roentgenographic appearance of the wrist.

A second potential but currently limited application of arthroscopy of the wrist is in the definitive treatment of noninfectious inflammatory synovitis. With the ad-vent of high-speed, constant suction/irrigation arthro-scopic shavers, synovectomy of the radiocarpal joint and to a limited degree the midcarpal joint can be performed arthroscopically. As a result of the arthroscopic exposure of the entire joint surface and internal capsule and syno-vial lining, one could argue the point that wrist arthros-copy may be the preferred procedure for roentgeno-graphic stages I and II rheumatoid arthritis. Morbidity associated with such a procedure would be low; postop-erative wrist mobilization could be initiated early; and the injury to soft tissue required for exposure of the ra-diocarpal joint significantly reduced. Both the midcarpal and radiocarpal joints would be amenable to arthro-scopic synovectomy.

Wrist arthroscopy for treatment of infectious synovitis of the wrist has generally not been used.

For primary bacterial infections of the wrist, arthrot-omy of the wrist with open synovectomy and copious irrigation of both the radiocarpal and midcarpal joints is the procedure of choice. Since the bacterial process often invades extensively into the wrist synovium and bone, it does not appear at the present time that arthroscopic synovectomy of the wrist would be an adequate surgical procedure in the face of overwhelming *Staphylococcus* or gram-negative sepsis. Irrigation of the wrist recom-mended for septic arthritis could be achieved quite readily arthroscopically using the two-portal or three-portal technique and could be considered in early pre-sentations of septic arthritis; possibly the addition of con-tinuous irrigation through arthroscopically placed drains or catheters would be sufficient for obtaining joint irriga-tion either alone or in combination with intraarticular antibiotics.

Patients with atypical mycobacterium involving the radiocarpal joint, tuberculosis of the radiocarpal joint, and a number of primary mycotic infections including sporotrichosis and coccidioidomycosis of the wrist have had wrist arthroscopy to assist or provide definitive diag-nosis. With a primary tuberculin or mycotic infection of the wrist synovium, synovectomy of the wrist performed arthroscopically could be a valuable procedure in reduc-ing the extent of the infectious process and assisting in antibiotic treatment (local lavage plus decreasing the size of the infectious inoculum). It is recognized that syno-vectomy alone is not adequate treatment for these dis-ease processes, but adequate synovectomy in combina-tion with appropriate chemotherapeutic agents could be of significant benefit in reducing the morbidity associ-ated with mycotic and tuberculin infections of the wrist.

In crystalline arthritis an arthroscopic washout may be helpful in controlling pain as well as in confirming the diagnosis.

In evaluation and treatment of rheumatoid arthritis involving the wrist, the primary goal is diagnostic biopsy followed by synovectomy as required of the radiocarpal, radioulnar, and midcarpal joints. The technique of wrist arthroscopy has been described in other chapters and need not be repeated here except to mention the peculi-arities of the arthritis patient, particularly the steroid-dependent rheumatoid arthritis patient. These patients may have very tender and brittle skin and severe finger deformities that will preclude the use of finger traps, even if one were to consider putting all five digits in the traps to more evenly distribute the load. Great care must be taken to prevent damage in these patients.

Our technique is to suspend the hand and wrist by overhead finger trap traction (sterile) with countertrac-tion across the midportion of the arm. The extremity is sterilely prepped, draped, and exsanguinated, and a tour-niquet is inflated. The arthroscopic technique starts by infiltrating the radiocarpal joint with 10 to 15 cc of nor-mal saline to distend the joint. A small arthrotomy is made just ulnar to the third extensor compartment adja-cent to the extensor pollicis longus tendon distal to Lister's tubercle. For inspection, a small (1.9-mm) arthroscope is inserted first. For diagnostic and therapeu-tic synovectomy, a 2.7- to 3-mm arthroscope is inserted with the arthroscope in place, and, using constant irriga-tion, the joint is inspected beginning at the scapholunate interval and moving first in a proximal and radial direc-tion toward the radial styloid and preradial styloid recess. Reversing the sequence, one can examine the articular cartilage of the scaphoid and scaphoid fossa of the distal radius, the scapholunate ligament interval, and the volar radioscapholunate ligaments. The lunate and lunate fossa of the distal radius are inspected, and the arthro-scope is advanced to the ulnar side of the wrist, where it is possible to examine the lunotriquetral joint and trian-gular fibrocartilage. A good evaluation of the ulnar side of the wrist from a radial portal may be difficult.

A second step in the procedure is to introduce a probe through the fourth dorsal portal or between the fourth and fifth dorsal portals with triangulation over to the ra-dial side of the wrist. Once again the synovium in the prestyloid recess of the distal radius, dorsal and volar wrist capsules, scapholunate interosseous ligament area, and volar recesses about the radioscapholunate ligament are examined. Through the ulnar portal, a small biopsy punch can be inserted and appropriate synovial biopsies obtained and sent to pathology for either fresh-frozen specimens, delayed permanent sections, or cultures.

When appropriate, synovectomy of the radial side of the wrist can be performed using a combination of small pituitary rongeurs, basket forceps, and small biopsy punch. An arthroscopic shaver with a constant suction irrigation system in place is inserted for synovectomy of the radial side of the wrist. In our experience there has been minimal difficulty in achieving a fairly complete synovectomy of the joint synovium through an ulnar approach, but a third arthrotomy between the first and second extensor compartments just at the distal tip of the radial styloid may be necessary to reach the volar radial capsule.

For debridement on the ulnar side of the wrist, the arthroscope is inserted through the fourth dorsal portal, and inspection of the ulnar side of the wrist is performed looking specifically for tears through the triangular fibrocartilage, tears of the lunotriquetrial ligament, and evaluation of synovitis involving the preulnar styloid recess. A combination of small biopsy punch, basket forceps, and arthroscopic shaver can be utilized to perform a synovectomy of the ulnar aspect of the wrist. It is usually necessary to perform a fourth arthrotomy for the insertion of debriding instruments through the dorsal L6 portal.

When there is advanced rheumatoid arthritis that involves central perforation of the triangular fibrocartilage and distal radioulnar joint, arthroscopic debridement including resection of the articular surface of the head of the distal ulna can be performed arthroscopically. This requires a combination of small ronguers as primary bone biting instruments in addition to the arthroscopic bur and arthroscopic shaver. This procedure can be tedious and in some circumstances is best performed open rather than by closed arthroscopic technique. Limited synovectomy of the distal radioulnar joint is a more preferable arthroscopic procedure, which can be performed through the central perforation of the triangular fibrocartilage.

In our experience, arthroscopic synovectomy of the midcarpal joint has not been necessary in rheumatoid arthritis. We prefer to inspect the midcarpal joint prior to synovectomy of the radiocarpal joint to avoid capsular distension, which might obscure examination of the midcarpal joint. It is quite reasonable, however, to anticipate quite adequate inspection of the midcarpal joint including the scaphotrapezial trapezoidal joint, scaphocapitate and lunocapitate articulations, and triquetrial hamate articulation by midcarpal arthroscopy. We have noted arthroscopically areas of cartilage damage both within the radial and midcarpal joint and keep this as part of the operative record.

At the completion of the synovectomy procedure, the tourniquet is deflated, thorough irrigation of the radiocarpal joint is performed, and 2 cc of cortisone is injected within the joint followed by closure of the arthrotomy portals. The extremity is then placed in a bulky dressing with a volar splint. The patient is given preoperative as well as postoperative antibiotics for a period of 24 hours. An orthoplast splint is then utilized for immobilization of the wrist for an additional period of 2–3 weeks.

RESULTS OF EVALUATION AND TREATMENT OF THE RHEUMATOID WRIST

We have used arthroscopy in more than 125 patients, 10 of whom had rheumatologic diseases involving the wrist. Our primary objective has been diagnosis, using the techniques described above. Of the positive diagnostic synovectomies, five wrists were treated by medical means alone, while the other five had operative synovectomy. In two patients, the synovectomy of the wrist was performed by arthroscopic techniques. In both cases the patient had mild to moderate rheumatoid synovitis. These cases demonstrate the ability of wrist arthroscopy to provide a thorough synovectomy of the wrist. When wrist arthroscopy was used for diagnosis only, the pathologists were able to identify inflammatory synovitis with rheumatoid granulation tissue response in all of the specimens, and we proceeded with operative synovectomy in the remaining three patients. To date, the arthroscopic synovectomy cases have not had recurrence of disease and did rehabilitate faster than did those who had operative synovectomy. The results are too recent to speculate whether the procedures will have long-term benefits and, in particular, whether arthroscopic synovectomy is preferable to open arthrotomy and synovectomy.

CONCLUSIONS

Arthroscopy of the wrist is beyond the investigational stage and currently represents an effective diagnostic and therapeutic technique for the treatment of inflammatory conditions involving the wrist. While its use in rheumatoid arthritis both diagnostically and therapeutically has been limited, in experienced hands it may prove to be more effective than open synovectomy. The arthroscopic surgeon can treat areas that are difficult if not impossible to reach through open arthrotomy. We have had experience in only two patients to date with mycotic infections involving the wrist in which arthroscopic procedures were helpful in defining the extent of radiocarpal and midcarpal joint involvement and in providing tissue for both pathologic and microbiologic analysis. We feel confident that such arthroscopy will be beneficial in the future and will aid our ability to both diagnose and potentially treat a number of inflammatory conditions involving the wrist with decreased morbidity and risk to our patients.

REFERENCES

1. Belsky MR, Feldon P, Millender LH, Nalebuff EA, Phillips C. Hand involvement in psoriatic arthritis. *J Hand Surg* 1982;7:203.
2. Chin Y-C. Arthroscopy of the wrist and finger joints. *Orthop Clin North Am* 1979;10:723–733.
3. Chin Y-C. Arthroscopy of the wrist joint. In Watanabe, M., ed. *Arthroscopy of Small Joints.* New York: Igaku-Shoin, 1985.
4. Dray GJ, Millender LH, Nalebuff EA, Phillips C. The surgical treatment of hand deformities in systemic lupus erythematosis. *J Hand Surg* 1981;6:339.
5. Ferlic DC. Inflammatory and rheumatoid arthritis. In: Lichtman DM, ed. *The Wrist and Its Disorders.* Philadelphia: WB Saunders, 1988.
6. Hastings DE, Evans JA. The lupus hand, a new surgical approach. *J Hand Surg* 1978;3:1979.
7. Moore JR, Weiland AJ. Gouty tenosynovitis in the hand. *J Hand Surg* 1985;10A:291.
8. Rodman GP, Schumacher R, eds. *Primer on the Rheumatic Diseases,* 8th Ed. Atlanta: Arthritis Foundation, 1983.
9. Rothfield NT. Systemic lupus erythematosis, clinical and laboratory aspects. In McCarty DJ, ed. *Arthritis and Allied Conditions.* 9th Ed. Philadelphia: Lea & Febiger, 1979.
10. Straub LR, Smith JW, Carpenter GK, Jr, Dietz GH. The surgery of gout in the upper extremity. *J Bone Joint Surg* 1961;43A:731.

Complications in Wrist Arthroscopy

Gary G. Poehling, M.D., *L. Andrew Koman*, M.D., *and David B. Siegel*, M.D.

Complications following arthroscopy are, fortunately, uncommon (1,4–7), and arthroscopy of the wrist is no exception. Most complications are avoidable with careful attention to correct portal use, with gentle handling of the articular cartilage, and with knowledge of the proper instrumentation.

ARTICULAR CARTILAGE DEFECTS

The most common complication following wrist arthroscopy is iatrogenic articular cartilage injury. It is most likely to occur during insertion of a cannula into the radiocarpal and midcarpal joints, and generally can be avoided with adequate wrist joint distraction and proper insertion of the instruments.

Distraction tension should be 5–10 pounds. When inserting an instrument into the radiocarpal joint, it is important to have the joint well distended and to follow the slope of the distal radius while applying a gentle twisting motion to the instrument. Once the tip of the instrument is inserted through the skin and subcutaneous tissue to the dorsal capsule, it is used to palpate the distal radius and the proximal carpal row before being inserted further into the radiocarpal joint. Similarly, the bones proximal and distal to the midcarpal joint are palpated before an instrument is inserted into the midcarpal radial portal. When establishing the midcarpal ulnar portal, each instrument should be inserted while under direct visualization through the midcarpal radial portal.

In general, partial-thickness articular cartilage injuries are not treated specifically, and they rarely cause significant postoperative disability. Larger articular cartilage injuries or flaps should be debrided to a smooth stable base as soon as they are recognized.

TENDON INJURY

Clinically significant extensor tendon injuries are extremely uncommon following wrist arthroscopy. Although there is the potential for extensor tendon injury every time an instrument is inserted, generally the tendons are lax enough so that the instrument being inserted will push them out of the way. A tendon injury is most likely to occur when the skin knife is inserted perpendicular to the tendon or when an instrument is inserted directly through the substance of a tendon. Most of the resulting injuries are partial-thickness tendon injuries and are not recognized clinically at the time they occur.

Strict adherence to standard portal entry and operative technique should prevent extensor tendon injuries. If such injuries have occurred, they will be manifested by an inability to extend the metacarpophalangeal joints fully after operation; the area should be explored through an open incision and the injuries repaired.

HARDWARE BREAKAGE

Pieces of hardware may be broken accidentally during operative wrist arthroscopy. Breakage is most likely to result from fatigue failure of the hardware with repeated use or the application of excessive force while steering the instrument through the contours of the wrist joint. Careful inspection of all instruments is mandatory preoperatively, especially the delicate basket forceps, which is the most likely to fail.

Power shaving instruments, debriders, and burs may shave the metal tip off the telescope, which creates metallic debris within the joint. These fragments must be washed out with irrigation of the joint to avoid subsequent abrasion of articular cartilage and chondrolysis.

VASCULAR INJURY

Injury to the radial artery in the anatomic snuffbox may occur with the use of the 1–2 portal or the STT portal. It is for this reason that we do not recommend use of these portals in routine wrist arthroscopy. To avoid a vascular injury in the 1–2 portal, the entrance should be dorsal in the 1–2 portal near the extensor carpi radialis longus tendon; for the STT portal, the entrance should be ulnar to the extensor carpi radialis longus tendon since the radial artery lies on the radial side of the tendon at that level.

With use of the other portals, a more common vascular injury is partial injury of one of the superficial veins in the dorsum of the wrist. Bleeding usually responds to direct pressure, but occasionally may require electrocoagulation.

Any excessive swelling in the postoperative area developing after deflation of the tourniquet should be considered a vascular injury and treated with direct pressure. If this fails to stop the bleeding, then exploration and vessel ligation or repair are indicated.

NERVE INJURY

The most devastating complication following wrist arthroscopy is injury to one of the subcutaneous nerves because that injury may lead to a reflex sympathetic dystrophy (2,3) (see below). Nerve injury can be avoided with strict adherence to technical detail. We have found injury to the superficial branch of the ulnar nerve to be most common with use of the 6U portal, and we therefore avoid that portal, using the 6R portal instead.

Nerve injury is recognized by loss of sensibility, and frequently pain, in a specific nerve distribution. Once a major nerve injury is recognized, it should be treated with operative exploration and repair. If repair is not possible, then the proximal nerve stump should be resected away from the zone of injury.

REFLEX SYMPATHETIC DYSTROPHY

Reflex sympathetic dystrophy may occur after known nerve injury, or after wrist surgery or wrist injury without a recognizable specific nerve injury. It is characterized by excessive (often burning) pain, impaired function, stiffness, and trophic changes. If unrecognized and/or untreated, reflex sympathetic dystrophy may resolve spontaneously or result in chronic pain and disability.

Unique Wrist Considerations

The anatomic characteristics of the wrist make it susceptible to a dystrophic response after arthroscopy. The sensory branches of the radial and ulnar nerves are subcutaneous and thus vulnerable to trauma. In addition, the deep, enclosed canals through which the ulnar nerve passes provide an environment conducive to compressive neuropathies, which may initiate and/or propagate a dystrophic response.

Neural Susceptibility

Sensory Nerves

The three sensory nerves of the wrist that are at greatest risk of triggering a dystrophic response following arthroscopy are the superficial radial nerve, the dorsal branch of the ulnar nerve, and the posterior interosseous nerve.

Iatrogenic laceration or contusion of the superficial radial nerve or one of its divisions during arthroscopy places the radial nerve at significant risk. Painful neuromas as well as a dystrophy may be produced.

The dorsal cutaneous branch of the ulnar nerve divides into two dorsal sensory branches, which are especially vulnerable during establishment of the 6U portal adjacent to the sixth extensor compartment for arthroscopy of the ulnar aspect of the wrist. It is for this reason that a portal adjacent to the radial side of the sixth extensor compartment (6R) should be used preferentially for ulnar-sided arthroscopic surgery of the wrist.

Posterior Interosseous and Posterior Antebrachial Cutaneous Nerves

Distal to the last motor branches to the extensor pollicis longus muscle, the posterior interosseous nerve continues adjacent to the third dorsal compartment to supply proprioception and sensibility to the wrist capsule and variable small areas of midline dorsal skin. Direct injury to the nerve from the arthroscopic telescope may cause persistent wrist pain and may trigger or exacerbate a dystrophic response.

Treatment

Prompt diagnosis and early intervention are important because early treatment of reflex sympathetic dystrophy is more effective than late treatment. Eighty percent of patients with reflex sympathetic dystrophy treated within 1 year of injury will show significant improvement in pain relief and restoration of function. Conversely, fewer than 50% of those treated after 1 year will show improvement. An unexpected degree of pain, a prolonged duration of pain, or a delay in recovery following injury or surgery may reflect a dystrophic process.

An initiating mechanical dystrophic focus of pain

should be sought and, if possible, corrected. For example, if a nerve has been cut, it should be repaired promptly. Operative correction of sequelae of the dystrophic event, such as arthrofibrotic joints, may be accomplished after appropriate treatment of the dystrophy. If operative release of these joints is warranted, measures to prevent recurrence of the reflex sympathetic dystrophy—such as continuous perioperative blocks or antisympatholytic agents—are recommended.

Physical Therapy

Physical therapy should be focused on prevention of atrophy and arthrofibrosis by the use of active and passive exercises and stress loading to counter the dystrophic phase and to aid in the recovery of the extremity. Mobilization to obtain maximal range of motion of the joint during anesthesia or under the protection of continuous or intermittent autonomic blockade may be useful. Physical therapy modalities such as transcutaneous nerve stimulators, contrast baths, and continuous passive motion machines may be used.

Oral Medications

Oral pharmacologic interventions are often effective in the management of reflex sympathetic dystrophy. Although the mechanisms of action of these medications are not completely understood, most involve reduction of sympathetic tone and/or improvement of nutritional blood flow to the involved extremity.

Stellate and Continuous Axillary Blocks

Sympathetic ganglion blocks may be used both for diagnosis and for the therapy of reflex sympathetic dystrophy, and they have been shown to provide excellent pain relief in selected patients. These blocks may be used serially over several months or years, and often provide permanent improvement in pain and functional disability. The blocks should be performed by experienced personnel and resuscitation equipment should be available. Our experience with combining a continuous sympathetic block for 5–7 days, an active and passive physical therapy program, and postblockade noninjectable oral pharmacologic medications has yielded favorable results in many instances.

REFERENCES

1. D'Angelo GL, Ogilvie-Harris DJ. Septic arthritis following arthroscopy, with cost/benefit analysis of antibiotic prophylaxis. *Am J Arthrosc Rel Surg* 1988;4:10–14.
2. Koman LA, Poehling GG. Reflex sympathetic dystrophy. In: Gelberman RH, ed. *Operative Nerve Repair and Reconstruction.* Vol. 2. Philadelphia: JB Lippincott, 1991, pp. 1497–1523.
3. Pollock FE Jr, Koman LA, Toby EB, Barden A, Poehling GG. Thermoregulatory patterns associated with reflex sympathetic dystrophy of the hand and wrist. *Orthop Trans* 1990;14:156.
4. Rames RD, Fox JM, Snyder SJ, Del Pizzo W, Friedman MJ, Ferkel RD. Arthroscopy: "No problem surgery." An analysis of complications of the next 2,388 cases [Abstract]. *Am J Arthrosc Rel Surg* 1990;6:160.
5. Small NC. Complications in arthroscopy: The knee and other joints. *Arthroscopy* 1986;4:253–258.
6. Small NC. Complications in arthroscopic surgery performed by experienced arthroscopists. *Am J Arthroscopy Rel Surg* 1988;4:215–221.
7. Sprague NF III. *Complications in Arthroscopy.* New York: Raven Press, 1989.

ELBOW

Elbow Arthroscopy

Introduction and Overview

Gary G. Poehling, M.D., *and Evan F. Ekman*, M.D.

Early anatomic studies suggested that the potential diagnostic and therapeutic benefits of elbow arthroscopy were far outweighed by the risk of injury to the nerves and arteries that surround the elbow joint (1). However, recent investigators have established safe portals of entry into the elbow joint (2,4,5,10), and this new understanding of arthroscopic portal anatomy, combined with the development of smaller instruments, has made elbow arthroscopy a viable alternative to open arthrotomy in the treatment of elbow disorders. Recent changes in patient positioning, refinement of equipment for small-joint arthroscopy, development of efficient irrigation systems, and establishment of a clearer definition of arthroscopic portals have been the primary contributions from recent investigators to elbow arthroscopy.

INDICATIONS

As a diagnostic tool, elbow arthroscopy provides information regarding the presence or absence of loose bodies, the condition of the synovium and intraarticular joint capsule, the quality of the articular cartilage, and any degree of instability. Patients with mechanical symptoms such as locking, periodic effusion, and painful range of motion in whom a graphic workup has failed to explain their symptoms and an adequate course of nonoperative treatment has failed to alleviate their symptoms are ideal candidates for operative elbow arthroscopy. The most common therapeutic indications for elbow arthroscopy are excision of osteochondral loose bodies; treatment of osteochondritis dissecans, synovitis, or chondromalacia; excision of marginal osteophytes; lysis of intraarticular adhesions; and adjunctive treatment of intraarticular fractures. The potential advantages of arthroscopy over open arthrotomy for the treatment of these conditions relate to the relative diminished morbidity associated with arthroscopic intervention compared with that of open incisions. In addition, arthroscopy provides a magnified view that is otherwise impossible without wide exposure of the joint.

PRONE TECHNIQUE

Patient positioning has emerged as one of the most important variables for a successful result from elbow arthroscopy (10). Although the supine position was initially advocated, it requires arm suspension with an overhead device and limits visualization of the posterior compartment. The prone position, recently advocated by Poehling and coworkers, allows the use of arthroscopic techniques that are standard in other joints, and it eliminates the need for traction devices, thus facilitating portal access and mobility of the joint (Fig. 1). The patient is placed prone after axillary block or general anesthesia is induced. Chest rolls are applied for padding and stability of the torso. An arm board with a sandbag is placed parallel to the operating table to maintain the brachium in a position parallel to the floor. Equipment such as the videocamera and recorder, motorized instrumentation, light source, and irrigation pump, is positioned

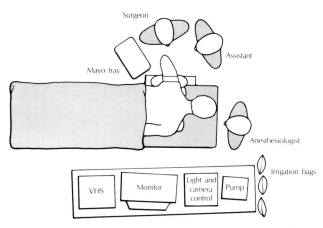

FIG. 1. Operating room setup for arthroscopy of the elbow, with the patient in the prone position.

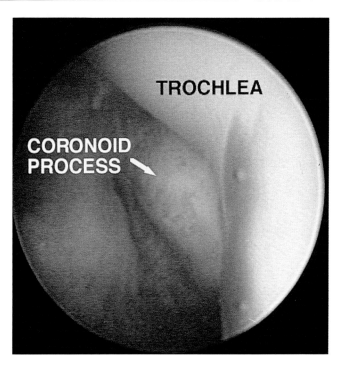

FIG. 2. View of the trochlea and coronoid process through the proximal medial portal.

on the opposite side of the patient (Fig. 1). Generally, a tourniquet is not used unless a pump is not available or excessive bleeding is expected.

The cutaneous landmarks are outlined for the olecranon, radial head, humeral epicondyle, and medial intermuscular septum. An 18-gauge needle is inserted into the anconeus triangle between the olecranon, radial head, and lateral epicondyle. Approximately 30 to 50 ml of lactated Ringer's solution is injected into the joint and the needle is withdrawn.

Portals

Three standard portals are used: the proximal medial, the anterolateral, and the posterolateral. The proximal

medial portal is used to visualize the anterior joint, including the trochlea, coronoid, medial condyle, radial head, and capitellum (Figs. 2 and 3). The anterolateral portal is used most often for instrumentation and operative intervention. The posterolateral portal is used primarily for visualization of the posterior joint, including the olecranon fossa and the tip of the olecranon.

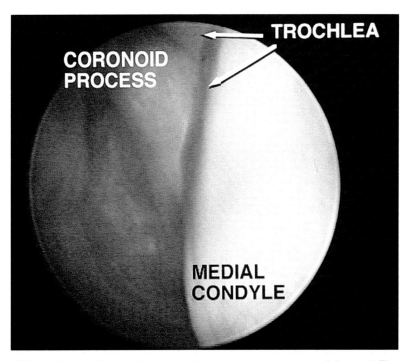

FIG. 3. View of the medial condyle through the proximal medial portal. The trochlea and coronoid process are in the background.

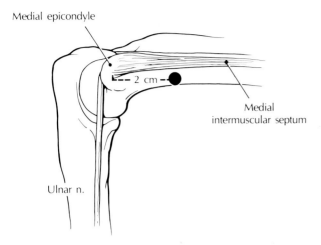

FIG. 4. The proximal medial portal is located 2 cm proximal to the medial epicondyle and anterior to the medial intermuscular septum.

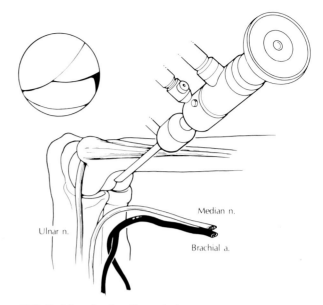

FIG. 5. Visualization through the proximal medial portal.

The proximal medial portal is located 2 cm proximal to the medial epicondyle and immediately anterior to the medial intermuscular septum (Fig. 4). To avoid injury to the medial brachial cutaneous and medial antebrachial cutaneous nerves, a longitudinal incision is made through the skin only. The sheath and blunt trochar for the standard 4.0-mm arthroscope are inserted along the anterior aspect of the medial intermuscular septum and the anterior surface of the distal humerus in direct contact with the bone, directing the tip toward the radial head (Fig. 5). During this entry, it is important to maintain contact with the intermuscular septum and the anterior humeral cortex to prevent injury to the median nerve and the brachial artery (Fig. 6). Entry into the joint is confirmed by a return of Ringer's solution through the cannula. A 30° arthroscope is inserted and the ante-

rior elbow joint can be clearly visualized. A pressure-monitoring outflow cannula is inserted through the anconeus triangle to ensure adequate flow distention and maintenance of intraarticular pressure during the procedure.

The anterolateral portal is established immediately anterior to the radial head, 1 cm distal to the radiocapitellar joint. This portal is established second, after the proximal medial portal is established. The telescope is removed from the proximal medial portal and a blunt rod is inserted through the sheath and directed anterolateral to the radial head (Fig. 7). It is important that the cannula be more lateral than anterior to the radial head to avoid injury to the posterior interosseous nerve. The

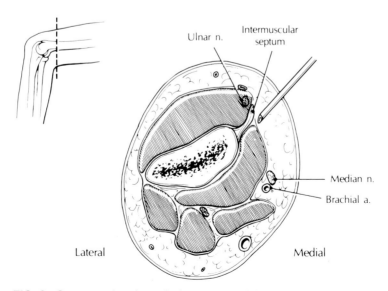

FIG. 6. Cross-section through the supracondylar region of the elbow demonstrating the relationships seen through the proximal medial portal.

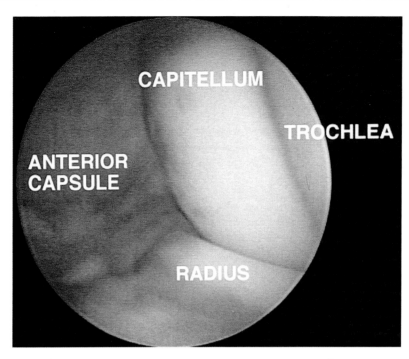

FIG. 7. View through the proximal medial portal. The position for the antero-lateral portal is easily seen anterior to the radial head in the anterior lateral capsule.

blunt rod is pushed through the anterolateral capsule into the subcutaneous tissue, and the skin is incised over the tip of the rod. A separate cannula is then inserted over the rod into the anterolateral aspect of the elbow joint.

For establishment of the posterolateral portal, the outflow pressure monitoring device is moved from its position in the anconeus triangle to the anterolateral portal. This spot in the anconeus triangle can now be used for telescope introduction and thus becomes the posterolat-

eral portal (Fig. 8). Visualization of the posterior joint is accomplished through this portal (Figs. 9–11).

In addition to the three described standard portals, a direct posterior triceps tendon-splitting approach may be used for inserting instruments in the olecranon fossa. A 5-mm incision is made 1.5 to 2 cm proximal to the tip of the olecranon process with the elbow flexed 90°. A blunt cannula and trocar are inserted into the olecranon fossa under direct visualization through a telescope in the posterolateral portal. Outflow and pressure monitoring are

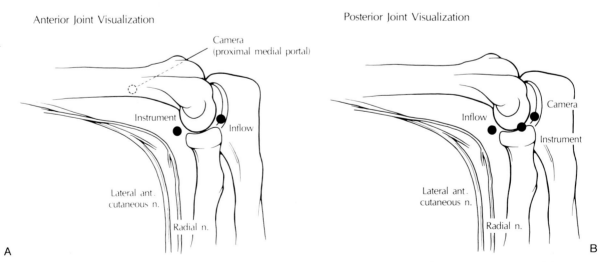

FIG. 8. A: View of the lateral portals as they are utilized during visualization of the anterior portion of the elbow. **B:** Lateral portals as they are utilized with posterior joint visualization.

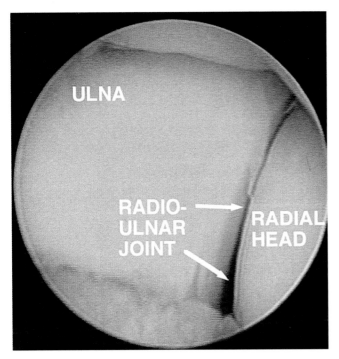

FIG. 9. View of the radioulnar joint through the posterolateral portal.

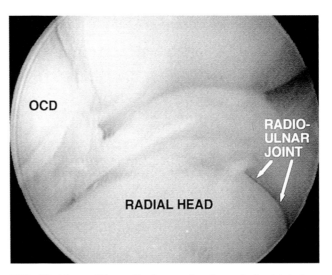

FIG. 10. View of the radioulnar and radiocapitellar joints in a patient with osteochondritis desiccans. This view is through the posterolateral portal.

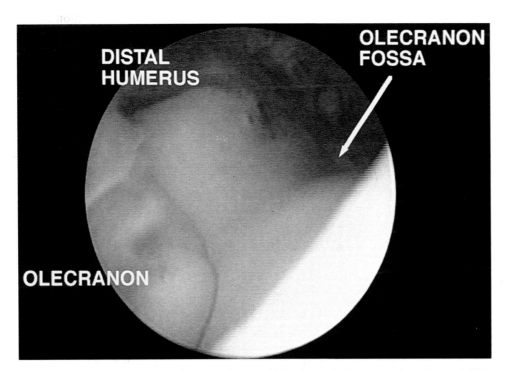

FIG. 11. View of the posterior olecranon humeral joint through the posterolateral portal. This view clearly demonstrates the olecranon fossa, the olecranon, and the distal humerus.

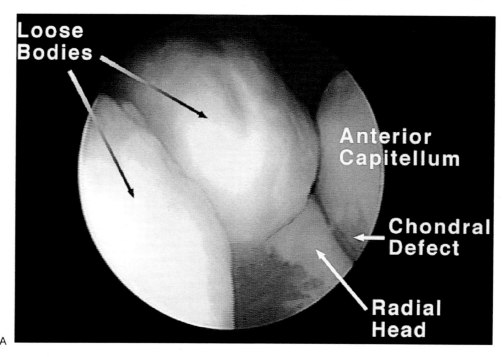

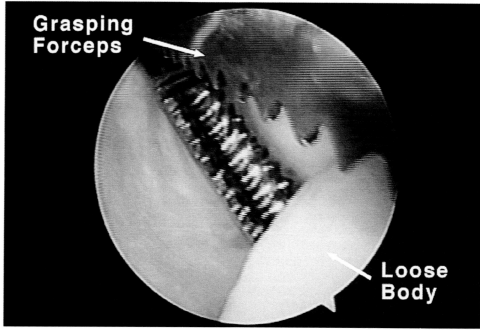

FIG. 12. **A**: View of the anterior joint through the proximal medial portal in an 18-year-old tennis player. Two large loose bodies are seen; in the background, a defect on the capitellum can be seen. **B**: Grasping forceps is used to remove one of the loose bodies through the anterior lateral portal.

maintained through the anterolateral portal during posterior instrumentation and visualization.

OPERATIVE ARTHROSCOPY

Synovectomy

Anterior synovectomy is accomplished with a telescope initially in the proximal medial portal and the synovial resector initially in the anterolateral portal. If necessary, these may be interchanged for complete anterior synovectomy. Posterior synovectomy is accomplished with the synovial resector in the posterior portal and the telescope in the posterolateral portal. Sutures are not used to close the portals, so fluid and blood can drain through the skin incisions. Postoperatively, motion is initiated as soon as the patient finds it comfortable.

Loose Bodies

Excision of loose bodies is an ideal indication for elbow arthroscopy (8,12,13). The use of suction basket forceps and Schlesinger grasping forceps facilitates removal of the loose bodies. For anterior loose bodies, visualization is accomplished through the proximal medial portal and the grasping forceps are inserted into the anterolateral portal (Fig. 12). For excision of posterior loose bodies, the posterolateral (telescope) and direct posterior (grasping forceps) portals are utilized (Fig. 13).

Arthritis

For excision of marginal osteophytes and removal of bone from the olecranon fossa, we have used both small and large burs. It is important that copious irrigation be used to remove any intraarticular bone that has been re-

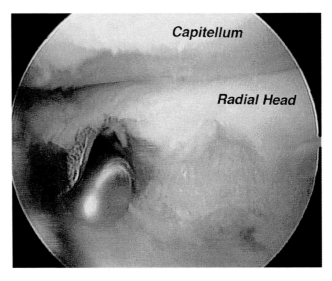

FIG. 14. Set-up for the initial phase of radial head excision. The telescope is in the proximal medial portal and the abrader is in the anterolateral portal.

sected from the margins of the joint. Arthroscopic fenestration of the olecranon fossa also has been used in the treatment of osteoarthritis (11).

Radial Head Excision

We have used arthroscopy for excision of the radial head, visualizing it through the proximal medial portal (Fig. 14). A large bur is placed into the anterolateral portal and the radial head is resected, including all articular cartilage and approximately 2–3 mm of the radial neck (Fig. 15). It is important to maintain the integrity of the

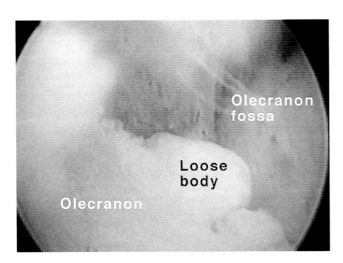

FIG. 13. View of the olecranon fossa with a loose body.

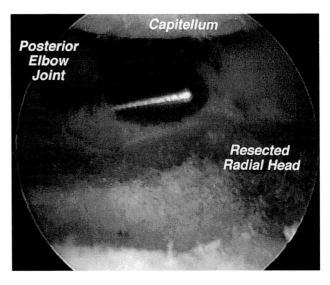

FIG. 15. The radial head resection is completed with the telescope in the anterolateral portal and the abrader in the posterolateral portal. A precise resection is possible, which minimizes postoperative morbidity.

annular ligament to prevent instability of the proximal radioulnar joint. Copious irrigation is used to clear the joint of all bony and cartilaginous debris. Full forearm rotation is observed under direct visualization to assure complete resection of the radial head. Postoperatively, a splint is worn for 3 days, after which active exercises are initiated.

Contracture

Capsular contracture also has been successfully treated with elbow arthroscopy (3,11). By releasing the proximal capsule and debriding the olecranon fossa, range of motion has been improved in pronation and supination, as well as in flexion.

COMPLICATIONS

Neurovascular injury is the most feared complication of elbow arthroscopy (6,9). Protective maneuvers include placing the patient in the prone position so that gravity can pull the anterior neurovascular structures (the median nerve and brachial artery) away from the joint space (10), and insuring full joint distension and elbow flexion to 90° before establishing the portals. Since the advent of use of the inside-out technique to establish the anterolateral portal, the risk of nerve injury has been significantly diminished. We have found that attention

to detail specifically related to the neurovascular structures has minimized the complication rate.

REFERENCES

1. Burman MS. Arthroscopy or the direct visualization of joints. An experimental cadaver study. *J Bone Joint Surg* 1931;13:669–695.
2. Carson WG Jr. Arthroscopy of the elbow. *Instr Course Lect* 1988;37:195–201.
3. Jones GS, Savoie FH III. Arthroscopic capsular release of flexion contractures (arthrofibrosis) of the elbow. *Arthroscopy* 1993;9: 277–283.
4. Lindenfeld TN. Medial approach in elbow arthroscopy. *Am J Sports Med* 1990;18:413–417.
5. Lynch GJ, Meyers JF, Whipple TL, Caspari RB. Neurovascular anatomy and elbow arthroscopy: Inherent risks. *Arthroscopy* 1986;2:190–197.
6. Marshall PD, Fairclough JA, Johnson SR, Evans EJ. Avoiding nerve damage during elbow arthroscopy. *J Bone Joint Surg* 1993;75B:129–131.
7. Norwicki KD, Shall LM. Arthroscopic release of posttraumatic flexion contracture of the elbow: A case report and review of the literature. *Arthroscopy* 1992;8:544–547.
8. O'Driscoll SW. Elbow arthroscopy for loose bodies. *Orthopedics* 1992;15:855–859.
9. Papilion JD, Neff RS, Shall LM. Compression neuropathy of the radial nerve as a complication of elbow arthroscopy: A case report and review of the literature. *Arthroscopy* 1988;4:284–286.
10. Poehling GG, Whipple TL, Sisco L, Goldman B. Elbow arthroscopy. A new technique. *Arthroscopy* 1989;5:222–224.
11. Redden JF, Stanley D. Arthroscopic fenestration of the olecranon fossa in the treatment of osteoarthritis of the elbow. *Arthroscopy* 1993;9:14–16.
12. Ruch DS, Poehling GG. Arthroscopic treatment of Panner's disease. *Clin Sports Med* 1991;10(3):629–636.
13. Ward WG, Anderson TE. Elbow arthroscopy in a mostly athletic population. *J Hand Surg* 1993;18A:220–224.

Imaging of the Elbow

Thomas L. Pope, Jr., M.D., *David B. Siegel,* M.D., *Gary G. Poehling,* M.D.,
and Michael Y. M. Chen, M.D.

The elbow is a complex articulation and may be involved by a variety of abnormalities. The major indications for arthroscopy of the elbow are loose bodies, posttraumatic sequelae, and inflammatory or synovial diseases. This chapter discusses the normal radiographic anatomy of the elbow, the range of diagnostic imaging techniques available to the arthroscopist for evaluation of this joint, and the radiographic findings of some of the more common pathologic entities for which arthroscopy is performed.

ANATOMY OF THE ELBOW

The elbow is a hinge, or ginglymus, joint composed of three distinct articulations: ulnohumeral, radiohumeral, and radioulnar. The ulnohumeral and radiohumeral components function as the hinge mechanism allowing flexion and extension; the radiohumeral and radioulnar components make possible the pivotal motions of pronation and supination. A common articular cavity incorporates the synovium, capsule, and ligaments, allowing the elbow joint to be considered a single anatomic element (75).

The distal end of the humerus flares into two articular surfaces: the capitellum, which articulates with the radial head, and the trochlea, which articulates with the coronoid process of the ulna. The distal humerus also expands into the medial and lateral condyles and epicondyles (Fig. 1).

The proximal ulna is composed of the olecranon posteriorly and the coronoid process anteriorly. The concave articular surface formed anteriorly between these anatomic components is called the semilunar or trochlear notch (51). A third articular surface contacting the cylindrical surface of the radial head is the radial notch, which also is present on the lateral side of the ulna. The proximal radius is primarily cylindrical. It has a concave superior surface and is constricted inferiorly at the radial neck (51). The prominent radial tubercle, the site of insertion of the biceps brachii muscle, is present distally and anteromedially (Fig. 2).

The flexor and pronator forearm muscles arise from the larger medial epicondyle, and the extensor forearm muscles from the smaller lateral epicondyle. The coronoid fossa anteriorly and the olecranon fossa posteriorly allow the full range of flexion and extension by providing a space for the coronoid and olecranon processes of the ulna during these excursions (Fig. 3).

The three major ligamentous groups within the elbow are the annular ligament, the ulnar collateral ligament, and the radial collateral ligament. The annular ligament is a thick, fibrous band attached to the anterior and posterior margins of the radial notch of the ulna. It forms a ring in which the proximal radius rotates, and it prevents inferior displacement of the radial head (Fig. 4). The ulnar collateral ligament has anterior and posterior compartments and a thick transverse band called the ligament of Cooper. The anterior and posterior bands arise

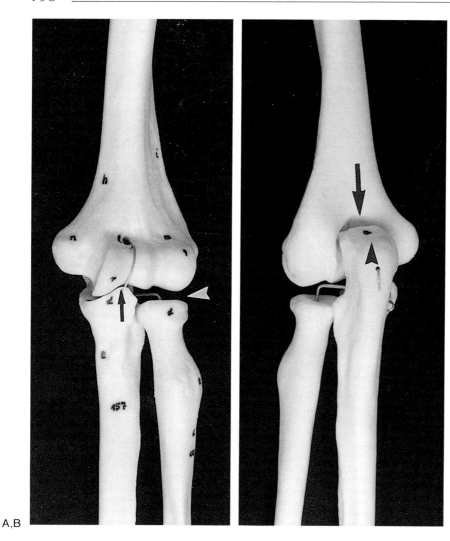

A,B

FIG. 1. A: Anterior view of the elbow of the skeleton shows flaring of the distal humerus into the medial and lateral epicondyles. Note the articulation of the coronoid process of the ulna with the trochlea (*arrow*) and the radial head articulation with the capitellum (*arrowhead*). **B:** Posterior view of the elbow shows the prominent olecranon fossa (*arrow*) and the olecranon process of the ulna (*arrowhead*).

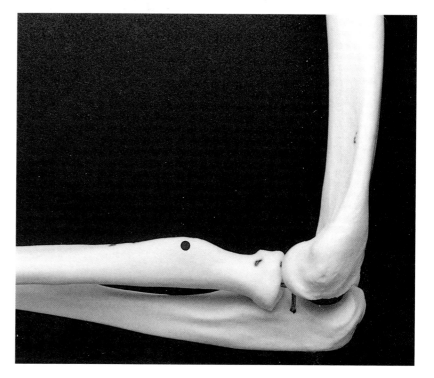

FIG. 2. Lateral view of elbow of the skeleton shows the prominent radial tubercle, site of insertion of the biceps brachii muscle (*black circle*).

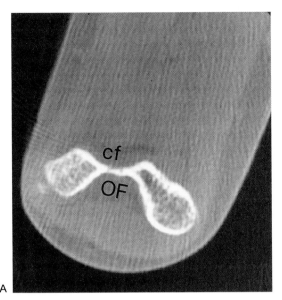 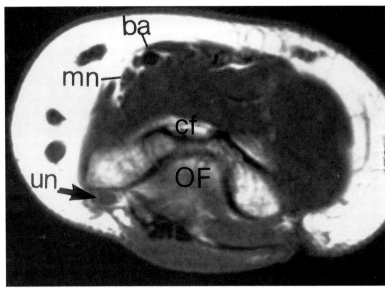

FIG. 3. A: Axial CT image of distal elbow showing the coronoid fossa anteriorly (cf) and the olecranon fossa posteriorly (OF). **B:** Axial MR scan at the same level as 3A shows the coronoid fossa (cf) and the olecranon fossa (OF) with the ulnar nerve (un), median nerve (mn), and brachial artery (ba). The major advantage of MR imaging is its soft-tissue contrast, which allows visualization of soft-tissue structures.

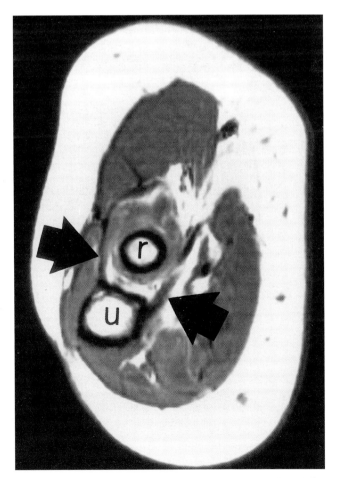

FIG. 4. Axial MR image shows the radius (r), ulna (u), and the ulnar insertion of the annular ligament (*arrows*).

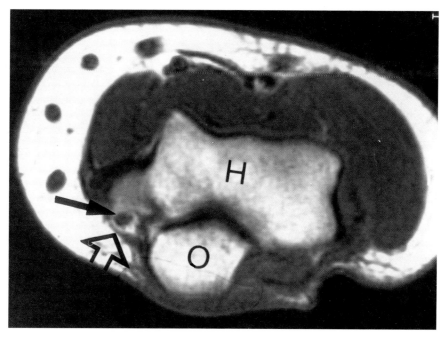

FIG. 5. Axial MR image shows distal humerus (H) and olecranon (O) with the ulnar nerve (*solid closed arrow*) and the ligament of Cooper (*open arrow*).

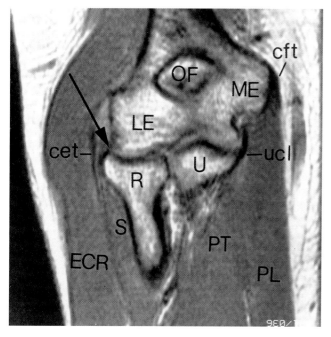

FIG. 6. Coronal T1-weighted MR image. LE, lateral epicondyle; ME, medial epicondyle; OF, olecranon fossa; R, radial head; U, ulna (coronoid process); ucl, ulnar (medial) collateral ligament; cet, common extensor tendon; cft, common flexor tendon; S, supinator muscle; ECR, extensor carpi radialis muscle; PT, pronator teres muscle; PL, palmaris longus muscle. *Long arrow* points to lateral collateral and annular ligaments.

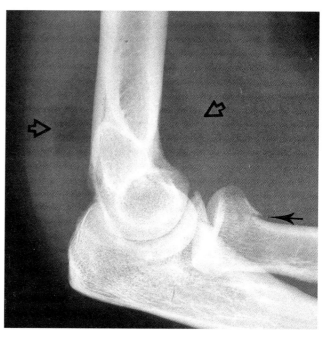

FIG. 7. Lateral plain film of the elbow shows radial head fracture (*closed arrow*) and large anterior and posterior fat pads (*open arrows*).

141

on the medial epicondyle and insert on the medial surfaces of the coronoid and olecranon. The ulnar nerve lies within fibrous tissue in the triangular space between these two components (Fig. 5). The ligament of Cooper stretches between the medial side of the olecranon and coronoid processes and unites the inferior ends of the anterior and posterior bands. The apex of the radial collateral ligament originates on the lateral epicondyle adjacent to and beneath the common origin of the extensor muscles; it flares distally to insert on the anterior and posterior margins of the radial notch of the ulna and onto the annular ligament (48) (Fig. 6).

The synovial capsule envelops fat anteriorly and posteriorly. These "fat pads" are important landmarks in assessing the elbow joint by plain radiography. The anterior fat pad normally is visible, but the posterior fat pad usually is hidden in the olecranon fossa of the distal humerus and can be seen only when the joint capsule is distended (8) (Fig. 7).

The anatomy of the muscles, vessels, and nerves of the elbow is complex (51). The ulnar and median nerves are probably the most important components to evaluate and can best be seen by magnetic resonance (MR) imaging (see Fig. 3B). Extensive descriptions of these anatomic relationships are available from other sources (75).

RADIOGRAPHIC TECHNIQUE AND ANATOMY

In discussing radiographic technique and anatomy of the elbow, a distinction must be made between the pedi-

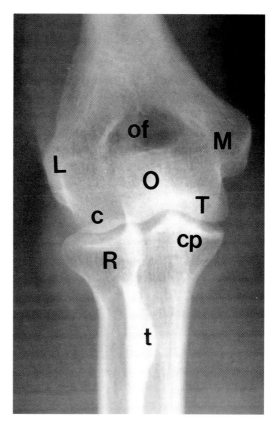

FIG. 9. AP view of the normal elbow. L, lateral epicondyle; M, medial epicondyle; O, olecranon process of ulna; of, olecranon fossa; c, capitellum; T, trochlea; R, radial head; cp, coronoid process; t, radial tuberosity.

atric and adult articulations due to the complex pattern of ossification in younger patients. The standard radiographic technique and anatomy of the adult elbow are described first.

Standard Elbow Radiographic Series in Adults

The routine radiographic elbow series consists of anteroposterior (AP), lateral, and oblique views. The AP view is best obtained with the patient seated at the radiographic table and the forearm fully extended and supinated on the radiographic cassette (Fig. 8). This maneuver helps to decrease the overlap of the proximal radius and ulna. The distal humeral condyles and shaft, the capitellum, the trochlea, and the proximal shafts of the radius and ulna can be seen well in this view. The olecranon of the ulna overlaps with the distal humerus and is not optimally visualized (Fig. 9).

On the standard AP radiograph, the valgus angle between the ulna and humerus is called the "carrying angle." Functionally, the carrying angle allows the hand to carry objects without their hitting the lateral aspect of the thigh. The carrying angle is measured by drawing

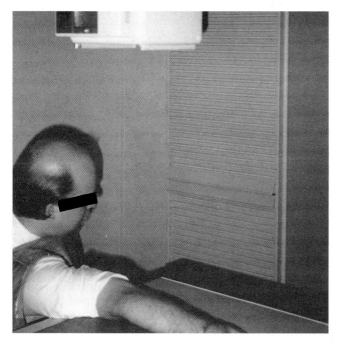

FIG. 8. Technique for obtaining AP view of elbow. Note that the palm is up.

lines parallel to the midportions of the distal humerus and proximal ulna (Fig. 10). The normal values for this measurement range from 2° to 26° (average 11°) in men and 1° to 22° (average 13°) in women (4). The AP radiograph also shows that the distal humeral articular surface is not perpendicular to the humeral shaft. This normal obliquity averages 83° in women (range 72–91°) and 85° in men (range 77–95°) (34,74).

The lateral view of the elbow is obtained with the arm flexed at 90° and the hand placed in neutral rotation parallel to the x-ray tube and perpendicular to the radiographic table (Fig. 11); the humeral epicondyles should overlap and should be perpendicular to the plane of the film (2). This projection demonstrates the distal humeral-olecranon articulation, the superior aspect of the radiocapitellum joint, and the shafts of the distal humerus, proximal radius, and proximal ulna. In the normal elbow, a line drawn through the midshaft of the humerus forms an angle of approximately 140° with the articular surfaces of the distal humerus; a line drawn parallel to the anterior humeral cortex, the "anterior humeral line," should pass through the middle third of the capitellum (58) (Fig. 12); and on both the lateral and AP views, a line bisecting the proximal radial shaft should pass through the capitellum (59) (Fig. 13).

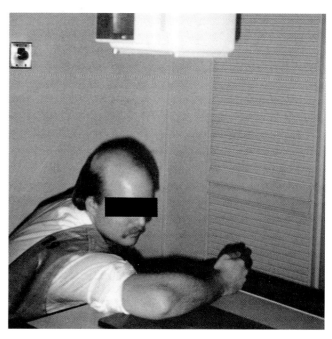

FIG. 11. Standard technique for obtaining lateral view of the elbow.

An important extrasynovial and intracapsular soft tissue structure, the anterior fat pad is normally seen in the lateral view and does not indicate abnormality (Fig. 14). The posterior fat pad, also extrasynovial and intracapsular, is not normally seen because it is hidden within the depression of the olecranon fossa. The posterior fat pad is seen only in pathologic states when the joint is dis-

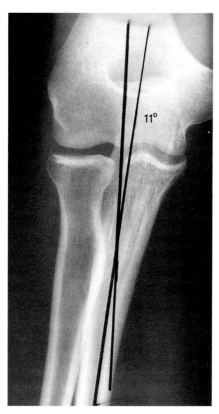

FIG. 10. "Carrying angle" of elbow. Lines parallel to the midportions of the distal humerus and proximal ulna show a carrying angle of 11°, which is normal.

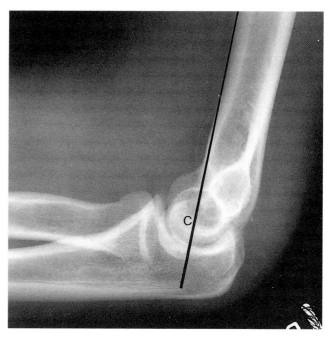

FIG. 12. Lateral view of elbow showing a line drawn parallel to the anterior portion of the humeral cortex normally passes through the middle third of the capitellum (c).

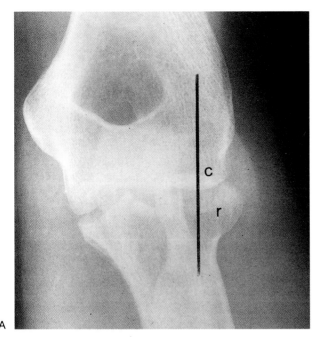
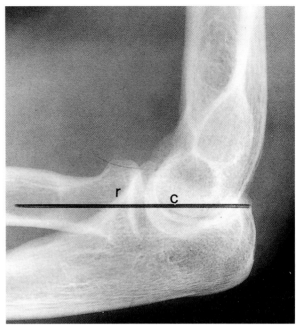

A   B

FIG. 13. AP (**A**) and lateral (**B**) views of the humerus show that a line bisecting the proximal radial shaft passes through the capitellum on both projections. This relationship is maintained regardless of the projection. c, capitellum; r, radial head.

tended by fluid or blood (8,9). In the setting of trauma, fracture of the radial head is the most likely cause of posterior fat pad distension (49,50) (Fig. 7). Lateral elbow radiography with a horizontal beam has been described as a way to demonstrate lipohemarthrosis (77) (Fig. 15).

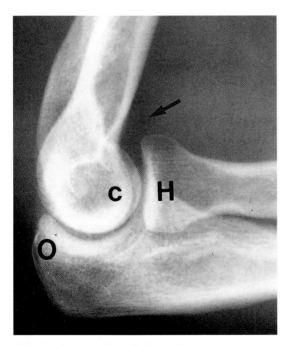

FIG. 14. Lateral view of elbow shows prominent anterior fat pad which by itself does not represent an abnormality (*arrow*). H, radial head; c, capitellum; O, olecranon.

Standard oblique views of the elbow are performed with the patient seated at the radiographic table and the arm fully extended. Filming is done in 45° of supination from the vertical and 45° of pronation from the vertical. These views show less overlap of the bony structures and different projections of the distal humeral cortex.

Supplemental Projections

A variety of projections to supplement the routine elbow series have been described. An axial projection with the elbow in acute flexion has been recommended for better visualization of the epicondyles, trochlea, groove between the medial epicondyle and trochlea, and olecranon fossa (36,60,71) (Fig. 16).

The cubital tunnel view as described by Wadsworth is useful for determining bony abnormalities contributing to ulnar compression neuropathy. This view is obtained with the elbow fully flexed and the humerus in external rotation. Tube centering is 1 inch distal to the point of the elbow (64,73) (Fig. 17).

The radial head–capitellum (R-H-C) view, first described by Greenspan and Norman in 1982 (27), has proved in some series to be helpful in demonstrating injury to the posterior aspect of the radial head, the coronoid process, and the capitellum (26–30,53) (Fig. 18). However, this projection should remain a supplemental one because recent studies reported that the R-H-C view alone does not show some radial head fractures that are demonstrated on the routine series.

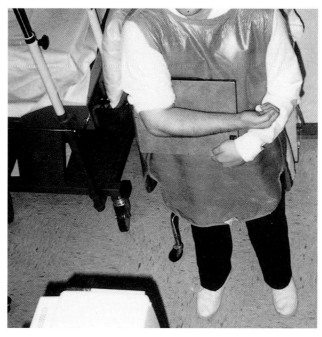

FIG. 15. Standard technique for obtaining a horizontal-beam lateral view of the elbow to demonstrate lipohemarthrosis.

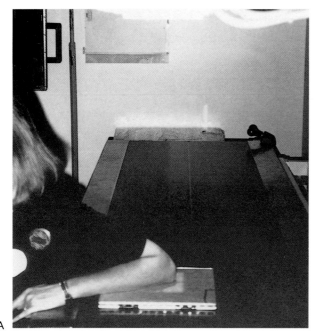

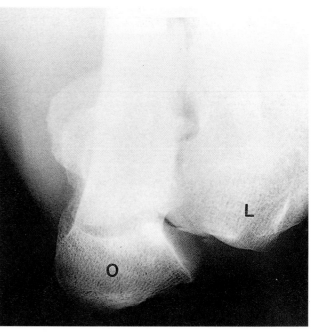

A

B

FIG. 16. A: Standard radiographic technique for obtaining axial view of elbow. **B:** Axial radiograph. O, olecranon; L, lateral epicondyle.

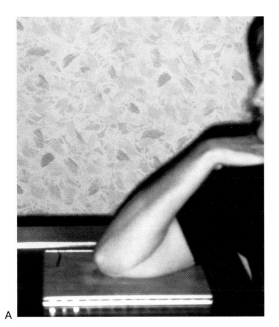

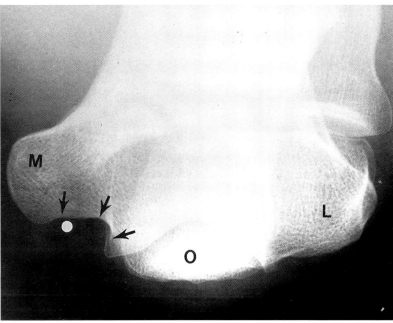

FIG. 17. **A:** Standard technique for obtaining the cubital tunnel view. **B:** Radiograph obtained showing the cubital tunnel (*arrows*). M, medial epicondyle; O, olecranon; L, lateral epicondyle. Location of ulnar nerve indicated by *solid white circle.*

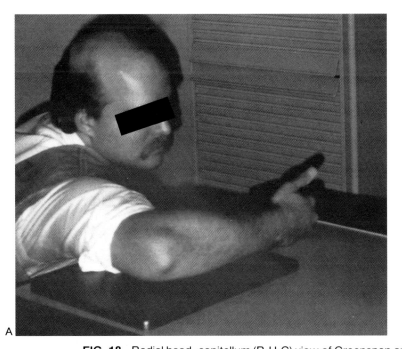

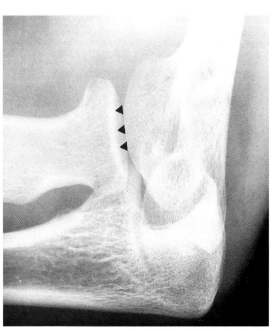

FIG. 18. Radial head–capitellum (R-H-C) view of Greenspan and Norman. **A:** Technique of obtaining the radial head capitellum view. **B:** Radiograph of the R-H-C view with excellent demonstration of the radial head (*arrowheads*).

Standard Elbow Radiographic Series in Children

The standard elbow series for the pediatric patient is the same as that used for the adult, but the appearance of the bones is different. The ages at which the ossification centers appear and their normal locations should be familiar to the arthroscopist.

The first epiphyseal ossification center to appear is the capitellum, which ossifies by the end of the first year of life. The progression is as follows: radial head (3–6 years), internal or medial epicondyle (5–7 years), trochlea (9–10 years), olecranon (6–10 years), and external or lateral epicondyle (11 years). CRITOE is a mnemonic commonly used to commit this information to memory.

The capitellum, trochlea, and lateral epicondyle fuse together around the time of puberty and merge with the lower humeral shaft at 17 years in boys and 14 years in girls. The medial epicondylar center fuses to the humeral shaft about a year later. The epiphysis of the olecranon process fuses to the ulnar shaft and the upper radial epiphysis fuses to the radial shaft at ages 15–17 years in boys and 14–15 years in girls (72).

FLUOROSCOPY

When the plain films do not answer the clinical question, fluoroscopy of the elbow may be indicated. An advantage of this technique is direct visualization of the osseous structures during motion, so that, potentially,

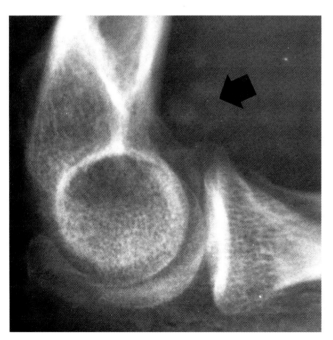

FIG. 19. Fluoroscopic spot film of patient 6 weeks after elbow dislocation shows irregular ossific densities anterior to the joint not well visualized on plain radiography (*arrow*).

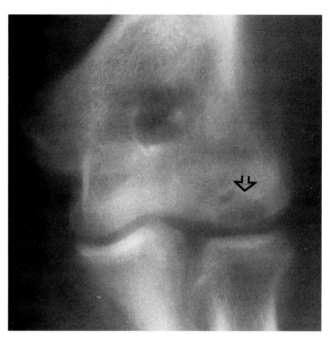

FIG. 20. Tomography of the elbow in patient with pain shows radiolucent subchondral defect in the capitellum representative of osteochondritis dissecans (*open arrowhead*). This lucency was much better appreciated on the tomogram than on the plain film.

minimally displaced fractures or fractures limited to one portion of the cortex can be seen. Fluoroscopy also is useful for identifying the exact location of calcifications that cannot be discerned from the plain radiographs (Fig. 19).

CONVENTIONAL TOMOGRAPHY

There are many overlapping osseous structures within the elbow joint. Because it is multiplanar, conventional tomography often is better for defining abnormalities than standard radiographic studies (Fig. 20), and it probably is most efficacious when combined with arthrography (20). However, due to the advantages of computed tomography, there are few current indications for conventional tomography.

COMPUTED TOMOGRAPHY

Computed tomography (CT) has distinct advantages over conventional tomography in the evaluation of the elbow. The axial anatomy of the elbow and radioulnar joints is demonstrated particularly well by this technique (16). Patients with acute or subacute pathologic conditions and those with flexion contractures can be studied adequately with CT (23,54). In almost half the patients in one study, CT provided information not available

TABLE 1. *Potential indications for elbow CT*

Severe or complex injuries
Suspected foreign body
Postdislocation (for intraarticular fragments)
Bony detail obscured by cast
Position of subtle fractures or dislocations in cast
Effusion on plain film without demonstrable fracture

From Franklin et al., ref. 23, with permission.

from plain radiographs, even though the additional information rarely modified therapy (23).

The major criteria for the use of CT in elbow studies are listed in Table 1. We use the technique primarily for evaluation of complex fractures, for better defining bony detail of arms in plaster casts, and for delineating injuries after dislocations. When combined with arthrography, CT also is an excellent diagnostic technique for difficult cases in the elbow (63) (Fig. 21). Three-dimensional CT is an exciting development that may prove to have applications in elbow imaging (39) (Fig. 22).

ARTHROGRAPHY

Arthrography of the elbow joint was first introduced in 1952. The major indications for this technique are outlined in Table 2 (1,7,37,60,65). Its common uses are

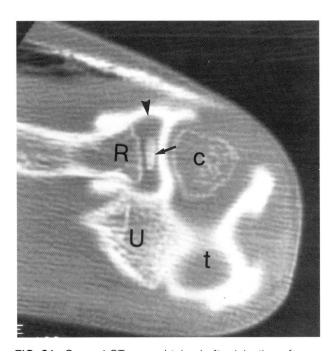

FIG. 21. Coronal CT scan obtained after injection of contrast demonstrates the ossified radius (R), ulna (U), and capitellum (c), and the nonossified ossification center of the trochlear (t). Note the central ossified portion (*arrow*) and the nonossified cartilaginous component (*arrowhead*) of the radial epiphysis.

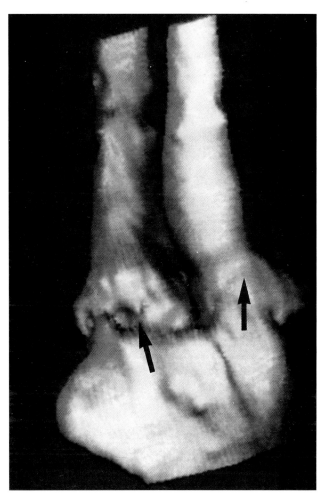

FIG. 22. Three-dimensional CT of the elbow shows olecranon and radial head irregularities after fracture (*arrows*).

for evaluating cartilaginous injury and for defining intraarticular loose bodies (7,65).

The single-contrast (contrast medium only) or double-contrast (contrast medium and air) technique can be used for arthrography of the elbow, although a number of published reports recommend the double-contrast method because it can be performed more quickly, its findings are easier to interpret, and it provides more detail than the single-contrast method (20,55,65). Usually, epinephrine is needed to retard contrast resorption, and

TABLE 2. *Potential indications for elbow arthrography*

Defining intraarticular loose bodies
Evaluating articular cartilage
Diagnosing capsular rupture after trauma
Locating calcifications seen on the plain film
Diagnosing synovial disease
Defining the location of juxtaarticular soft-tissue masses
Demonstrating elbow joint confines
Documenting needle position for arthrocentesis

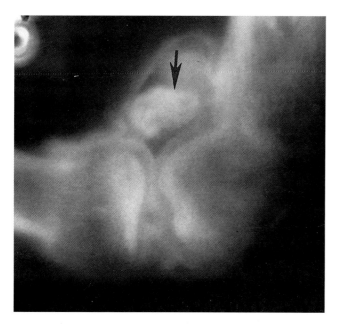

FIG. 23. Lateral tomogram of double-contrast arthrogram shows ossific fragment ("loose body") within the joint (*arrow*). (Courtesy of Dr. Art Newberg, New England Baptist Hospital, Boston, MA.)

most elbow arthrograms should be combined with linear tomography or CT for best results (20,63) (Figs. 21 and 23).

ULTRASOUND

Some investigators have advocated ultrasonography for examining the elbow because it is inexpensive and quick (3). The major indications reported for elbow sonography are effusions, fat pads, and loose bodies (24,35,42,61).

MAGNETIC RESONANCE IMAGING

Magnetic resonance (MR) imaging, because of its superb inherent soft-tissue contrast, is an excellent adjunct technique for diagnostic evaluation of the elbow (5,6,13,14,38,41). For best results, a small field of view should be used. Dedicated extremity coils are needed, and the elbow, as any other anatomic structure, should be placed as near as possible to the center of the magnet. As with other joints, the site of specific tenderness should be marked on the skin with a calgon bead or other lipid-containing material that can be imaged easily by the scanner. After an axial scout view to localize the elbow, standard T1-weighted and T2-weighted or T2*-weighted (gradient-recalled echo) images are performed in the axial, coronal, and sagittal planes. The scan can then be tailored to the clinical situation with other imaging ori-

TABLE 3. *Indications for elbow MR imaging*

Tendon injuries
Ligament injuries
Nerve entrapment syndromes
Trauma to the immature skeleton
Osteochondral injuries
Osteochondritis dissecans
Avascular necrosis
Inflammatory conditions
Soft-tissue masses/neoplasms
Primary osseous neoplasms
Subtle bone marrow abnormality

entations. Intravenous contrast enhancement may be helpful in diagnosing soft-tissue mass lesions, but its efficacy is still investigational. MR imaging of the normal anatomy of the elbow has been described in two recent publications (14,41), but the usefulness of MR imaging in delineating pathologic processes in the elbow in a large series of patients has not been reported.

The major indications for elbow MR imaging are shown in Table 3. MR imaging should be used only as an adjunct imaging procedure when indicated by the clinical history, physical examination, and plain radiographs. Consultation between clinician and radiologist is imperative for the best diagnostic management.

PATHOLOGIC PROCESSES OF THE ELBOW

The major categories of disease in the elbow that are relevant for arthroscopists are sequelae of trauma (either acute or chronic), synovial disease, and inflammatory or neoplastic conditions. As with any other joint, the plain radiograph is the first imaging test to obtain after a careful history and physical examination are completed. The findings on the plain film will then help to direct the imaging workup before any arthroscopic or surgical therapy.

Sequelae of Acute Trauma

Fractures of the Radial Head and Neck

The most common fractures of the elbow occur in the radial head or neck, and result from axial and valgus forces produced by a fall on the outstretched arm. Other common injuries include capitellar or medial collateral ligament damage, fractures of the distal radius, distal radioulnar joint injury, or damage to the articular cartilaginous regions (45,56,67).

Acute fractures of the radial head usually are associated with point tenderness. Routine radiographic findings of radial head fracture include a posterior fat pad

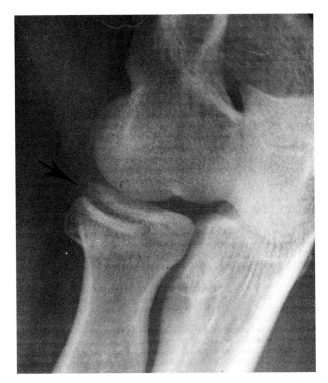

FIG. 24. Oblique view of left elbow after fall shows displaced fracture of the radial head (*arrow*).

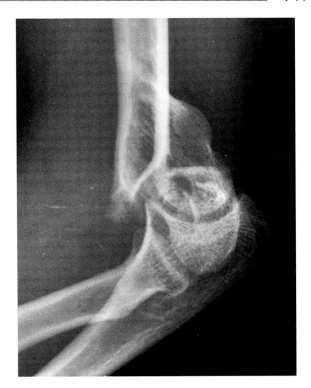

FIG. 25. Lateral view of the elbow shows a supracondylar fracture with marked posterior displacement of the distal humeral fragment.

sign, discontinuity of the cortical surfaces or trabecular pattern of the radial head, displacement of the proximal radial head fragment in cases of severe fracture, or sclerosis at the site of an impacted fracture (57) (Fig. 24). Subtle nondisplaced radial head fractures may require CT or MR imaging to confirm (23,54). However, a patient with an acute injury and plain films of the elbow showing a positive posterior fat pad sign and no detectable bony abnormality should be presumed to have a nondisplaced radial head fracture until proved otherwise.

The radial neck is usually extracapsular, and isolated fractures at this site may not displace the fat pads (62).

Supracondylar Fractures

Fractures of the supracondylar segment of the humerus are the most common sequelae of acute elbow trauma in the child (52). Two major types of injuries occur, depending on the mechanism of injury. Falling on the outstretched arm with forced hyperextension of the elbow results in posterior displacement of the distal humeral fragment (Figs. 25 and 26). Usually, in these cases the anterior humeral line is abnormal and the posterior fat pad may be displaced (22). Baumann's angle, the angle subtended between the axis of the humerus and the lateral condylar (capitellum) growth plates, which nor-

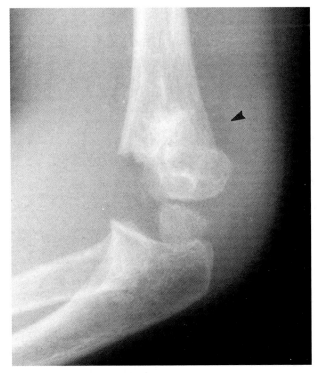

FIG. 26. Lateral view of elbow of 3-year-old child shows a supracondylar fracture with posterior displacement of the distal fragment and a posterior fat pad sign (*arrowhead*).

mally is about 75°, also may be abnormal (17). Less commonly, axial loading on the flexed elbow or an anteriorly directed force to the olecranon may result in anterior displacement of the distal humeral fragment (17,56).

CT may be practical in the patient with supracondylar fracture for detecting the axial rotation and angulation of the epiphyseal fragment (usually of the cubitus varus type) (31).

Growth Plate and Epiphyseal Injuries

Before the epiphyses close, injuries to the nonossified chondroepiphyseal centers may be difficult to diagnose by plain radiography. The most common pediatric injuries to the elbow are homologues of the acute injuries in the adult. Examples include supracondylar humeral fracture in the older child and the Salter–Harris type I injury in the infant, and condylar fractures of the adult and Salter–Harris types III and IV injuries of the medial (trochlear) and lateral (capitellar) chondroepiphyses of the child (Figs. 27 and 28). In all these injuries, comparison films of the opposite elbow with similar positioning and technique are important in arriving at a diagnosis (56). Alternative diagnostic techniques include arthrography and MR imaging. However, in childhood acute injuries, these techniques are extremely difficult to perform due to the patient's pain.

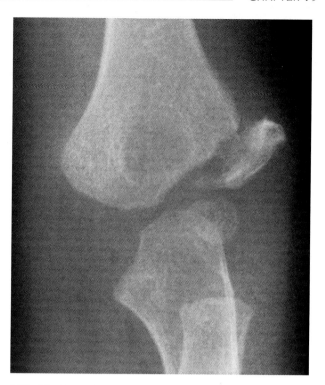

FIG. 28. Lateral condyle fracture: AP view of the elbow shows a fracture of the lateral condyle with lateral displacement of the distal fragment.

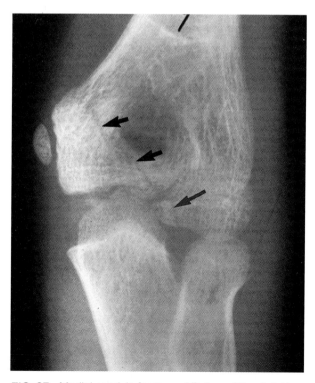

FIG. 27. Medial condyle fracture: AP view of the distal humerus in 9-year-old child shows a nondisplaced Salter–Harris type IV fracture (*arrows*) through the medial condyle (Kilfoyle type I).

Avulsion Injuries

In the child, the traction of strong soft-tissue attachments on the relatively weak elbow apophyses during acute or chronic repetitive trauma may result in avulsion injuries. These injuries account for approximately 10% of elbow fractures in children (17,56). The most common avulsion injury is separation of the medial epicondylar apophysis. This usually is caused by a fall on the outstretched hand or on the elbow (15). The best known of the medial epicondylar avulsion injuries, however, is the little leaguer's elbow, seen in young baseball players. This avulsion fracture of the medial epicondylar apophysis is caused by the tug of the flexor pronator group of muscles during the acceleration phase of throwing (12).

Familiarity with the ossification pattern of the distal humerus is necessary to diagnose this injury. The medial epicondyle ossifies between the ages of 5 and 7 years. It should lie in close proximity to the shaft of the humerus. With avulsion, the radiograph shows overlying soft-tissue swelling and displacement of the ossification center (12,18,25) (Fig. 29). In subtle cases, comparison with the asymptomatic normal side also may be important in making this diagnosis. Arthrography or MR imaging can show fractures of the nonossified chondroepiphyseal centers, but it is not used often to diagnose this condition because the clinical signs are relatively specific with the correct historical information. Although most com-

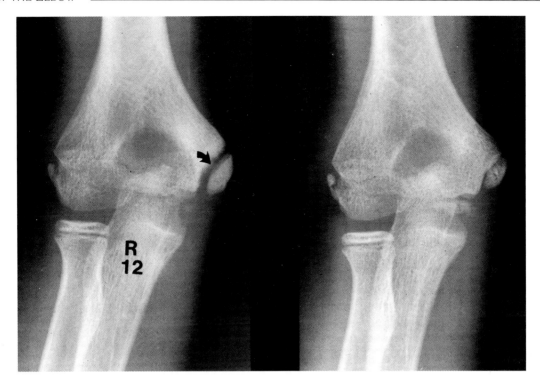

FIG. 29. Avulsion fracture of medial epicondyle (*curved arrow*) of right elbow of 12-year-old child (little leaguer's elbow). The normal left elbow is shown for comparison. (Courtesy of Dr. Art Newberg, New England Baptist Hospital, Boston, MA.)

monly an acute fracture, this injury may be more chronic and insidious; in such cases the radiographic findings include separation, fragmentation, enlargement, or roughening of the medial epicondyle (68).

Elbow Dislocations

Dislocations at the elbow are common injuries. Radial head dislocations occur with fractures of the proximal ulnar shaft from a fall on the dorsal part of the forearm. This injury is part of the Monteggia fracture–dislocation complex (58). The ulnar fracture usually is angled anteriorly and, in children, may be a bowing or greenstick-type fracture without a distinct fracture line (10). The diagnosis is best made on the lateral projection (Fig. 30).

Elbow dislocations most commonly result from a fall on the outstretched arm causing posterior and lateral displacement of the radius and ulna. In adults the coronoid

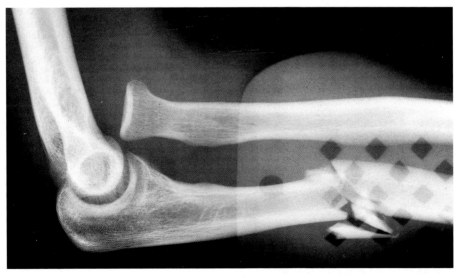

FIG. 30. Lateral view of the elbow shows fracture of the midportion of the ulna with superior displacement of the radial head (Monteggia fracture).

process of the ulna or radial head may be fractured, and in children the medial epicondylar ossification center may be avulsed and entrapped during reduction (15,58) (Fig. 31).

In cases of chronic dislocation, ancillary arthrography may be helpful in demonstrating the primary ligamentous injury, identifying the capsular laxity, and showing intraarticular fragments (46). MR imaging may be an alternative procedure in these patients.

Complications of Fracture/Dislocation

Potential sequelae of elbow fractures and dislocations include contractions, osteochondral fragments, myositis ossificans, capsular calcification, and nerve injury. Contractions are clinical diagnoses, and the radiographic findings may be minimal. Osteochondral fragments, or "loose bodies," may be shed into the joint and become nidi for the deposition of concentric layers of cartilage, which then may calcify. Nourished by the synovial fluid, the cartilage may continue to grow and produce masses that can restrict elbow motion (44). Heavily calcified loose bodies may be diagnosed by plain radiography (Fig. 32), or arthrography (with or without CT) may be necessary (Fig. 33) (23,55,63,65). Usually no more than

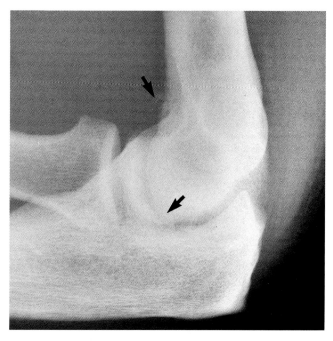

FIG. 32. Lateral view of elbow in patient with osteochondritis dissecans of the capitellum shows ossified intraarticular bodies (*arrow*).

three osteochondral bodies are formed by trauma, in contrast to the numerous fragments seen in synovial chondromatosis.

Myositis ossificans (posttraumatic soft-tissue ossification) occurs in approximately 3% of elbow injuries and most commonly is seen after elbow dislocations (66).

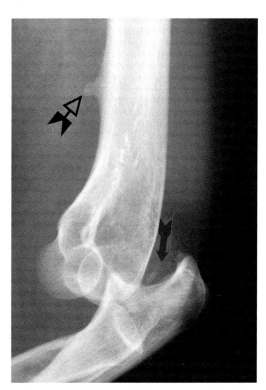

FIG. 31. Lateral view of the elbow of a patient who fell against a wall shows posterior dislocation of the elbow. Note the intraarticular fragments (*closed arrow*). A normal variant of the supracondylar process is demonstrated by the *open arrowhead*.

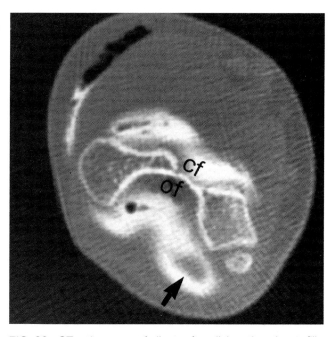

FIG. 33. CT arthrogram of elbow after dislocation shows filling defect within the contrast representing a nonossified intraarticular loose body (*arrow*). cf, coronoid fossa; of, olecranon fossa.

Hemorrhage into the soft tissues and mobilization of the joint are thought to contribute to the formation of myositis ossificans (Fig. 34). Capsular calcification, presumably caused by bleeding into the synovial membrane, also can be seen after elbow injuries.

Injuries to vessels and nerves may result from elbow fractures or dislocations. Acute vascular injury is treated with surgery, and in certain cases arteriography may be required. Chronic pain or disability that cannot be evaluated well clinically may be evaluated with MR imaging because the inherent soft-tissue contrast of the technique makes it possible to image vessels, nerves, and tendons.

Osteochondritis(osis) Dissecans of the Capitellum (Panner's Disease)

Osteochondritis(osis) dissecans is a type of avascular necrosis seen in many anatomic sites; most likely it is caused by trauma. Acute or chronic repetitive injury causes a series of events including trabecular micro- or macrofractures, diminished vascularity, hypoperfusion, and eventually osteonecrosis of bone. In the early stages of the process, articular cartilage covers the osteonecrotic bone. However, with continued trauma, the articular cartilage and cortex may be destroyed. The resulting fragment of bone may stay attached to its donor site, or it may fall into the joint as one or more free fragments (40).

Osteochondritis dissecans has a predilection for convex surfaces; in the elbow it is most commonly seen in the capitellum (47,76). Plain films show an ovoid lucency within the capitellum, possibly surrounding a dense, round, bony fragment (Fig. 35). The most important diagnostic information in determining therapy is the integrity of the articular cartilage surrounding the bony defect. CT-arthrography has proven to be of value in determining the status of the articular cartilage and any other associated intrasynovial abnormality (11,32). There may be a future role for MR imaging in osteochondritis dissecans of the capitellum in view of the proven value of the technique in evaluating the knee for the same disease (19).

Tendon Injuries

Isolated acute tears of the tendons at the elbow joint are unusual. The more common tears are in the biceps and triceps tendons. Usually, these injuries are diagnosed clinically and imaging is not required. When imaging is necessary, MR imaging is the best available method to determine the degree of tendon injury preoperatively.

"Tennis elbow," a syndrome of disabling lateral elbow pain, particularly with active extensor muscle contraction, is a commonly encountered entity in young and middle-aged adults involved in sports activities that require frequent rotatory motion and extension of the forearm (70). The plain films may show periostitis at the insertion of the common extensor tendon in patients with chronic symptoms. MR imaging is the best means of

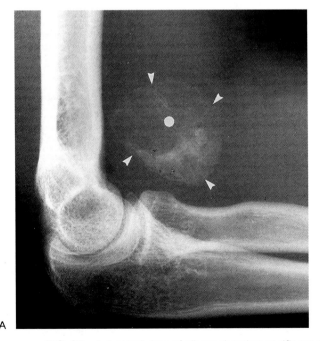
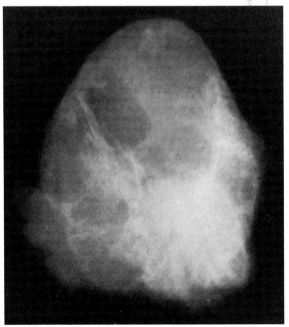

A
B

FIG. 34. A: Lateral view of elbow showing ossific mass in soft tissues anterior to elbow. Note the heavily ossified rim (*white arrowheads*) and the lucent center (*solid white circle*) characteristic of myositis ossificans. **B:** Radiograph of surgical specimen in same patient after removal.

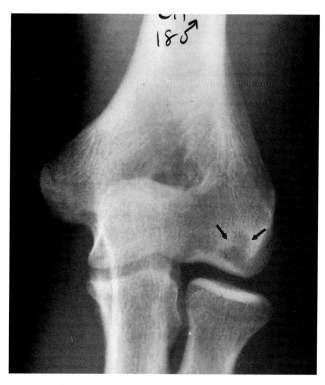

FIG. 35. Oblique view of the elbow shows radiolucent defect in the subarticular area of the capitellum representative of osteochondritis dissecans (*arrows*).

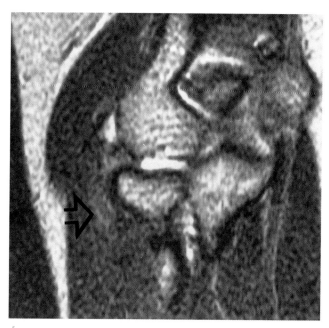

FIG. 36. Coronal T2-weighted MR image of a patient with symptoms of tennis elbow shows slightly increased signal intensity in the region of the common extensor tendon adjacent to the lateral epicondyle representing edema within the soft tissue (*open arrow*).

demonstrating the soft-tissue signs of this disorder. Increased signal intensity in the proximal portions of the common extensor tendon adjacent to the lateral epicondyle on T2-weighted or gradient-echo images represents edema in this region (Fig. 36). Fluid collections within or beneath the tendon also may be seen (21). MR imaging may provide concrete evidence for assessing the resolution of the disease.

Sequelae of Chronic Trauma

Calcific Tendinitis

Calcific tendinitis is characterized radiographically as calcification within the substance of tendons. The most common causes of tendinitis are (a) chronic repetitive trauma that results in micro tears, followed by repair and dystrophic calcification, and (b) age-related degeneration of the collagenous structure of the tendon. Tendinous calcification also can be seen in enthesopathic disorders such as diffuse idiopathic skeletal hyperostosis (DISH, Forestier's disease) and the seronegative spondyloarthropathies.

The plain-film diagnosis of calcific tendinitis is made by the demonstration of thin linear calcifications within a tendon. Generally, no other imaging studies are needed to make this diagnosis (Fig. 37).

Spur Formation

Spur formation in the elbow may be seen in osteoarthrosis or as a sequela of acute or chronic trauma. Degenerative olecranon spurs near the attachment of the triceps muscle also are common causes of elbow disabil-

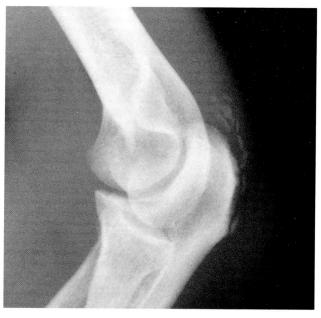

FIG. 37. Slightly oblique view of elbow showing multiple linear calcifications within the triceps tendon representing calcific tendinitis. (Courtesy of Dr. Stanley Bohrer, Bowman Gray School of Medicine, Winston-Salem, NC.)

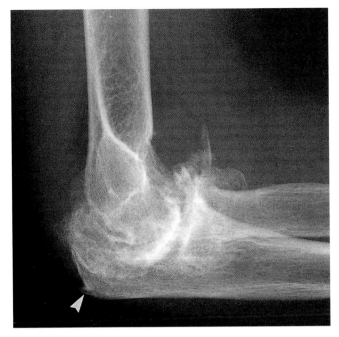

FIG. 38. Lateral view of elbow showing marked degenerative change of the elbow with a small olecranon spur (*white arrowhead*).

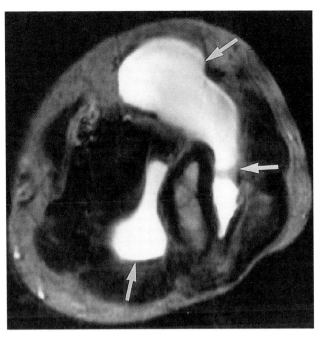

FIG. 39. Axial T2-weighted MR image in a patient with septic arthritis shows large joint effusion (*white arrows*).

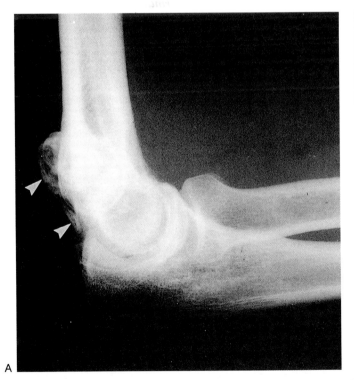

A

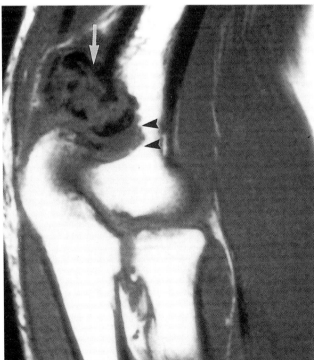

B

FIG. 40. Synovial chondromatosis. **A:** Lateral plain film of the elbow shows ossific densities in the olecranon fossa (*white arrowheads*). **B:** Sagittal T1-weighted MR scan confirms large osteochondral loose body (*white arrow*) with erosion of the olecranon fossa (*black arrowheads*).

ity in the middle-aged and elderly. These bony excrescences may be seen in younger patients as a result of valgus extension overload syndrome, which most commonly is seen in baseball pitchers (18).

The diagnosis of olecranon spur formation is made easily with routine plain films (Fig. 38). Degenerative changes also can be seen in other regions, such as the radial head–capitellum. Imaging with CT and MR is rarely needed in this setting unless the exact site of the spur cannot be determined from the plain films.

Synovial/Bursal Disease

Joint Effusion

The normal elbow contains a small amount of fluid within the capsule of the joint. Excessive fluid or hemorrhage within the elbow is seen most commonly with intraarticular fracture or with inflammatory processes such as infections or arthropathies. The effusion can be detected on plain films by the displacement of the anterior and posterior fat pads (Fig. 7). MR imaging also exquisitely demonstrates an effusion as a distension of the capsule. The fluid is best seen as high signal intensity on T2-weighted or gradient-echo images (Fig. 39). As previously noted, MR imaging has the additional advantage of demonstrating articular cartilage and bone marrow.

Synovial Chondromatosis

Synovial chondromatosis is a disorder of unknown etiology manifested by metaplasia and hypertrophy of the synovium. Villous projections from the synovium or from articular cartilage shed into the joint, where they become nidi for cartilaginous growth. Characteristically, multiple calcified loose bodies of varying sizes and shapes may be seen on plain radiographs (Fig. 40A). CT-arthrography and MR imaging are adjunctive imaging tests to diagnose this disorder (43,69) (Fig. 40B).

Other Inflammatory and Neoplastic Conditions

A variety of inflammatory and osseous or soft-tissue neoplastic conditions may occur at or near the elbow. In general, evaluation of these diseases should begin with plain radiography. MR imaging is the next best procedure for determining the intramedullary and soft-tissue extent of a lesion. CT also may be helpful in showing an intramedullary or soft-tissue matrix that is not well delineated by plain films.

In summary, the elbow should first be evaluated by plain radiography, and the choice of the appropriate adjunct imaging tests should be based on the history and physical examination. Close cooperation and communication between the clinician and the radiologist are important for optimal patient care.

ACKNOWLEDGMENTS

The authors appreciate the excellent administrative assistance of Angela Overby, Donna Garrison, and Nancy Ragland. The technical assistance of John Cassell, Dennis Daniels, and Rita Lee is also greatly appreciated.

REFERENCES

1. Arvidsson H, Johansson O. Arthrography of the elbow joint. *Acta Radiol* 1955;43:445–452.
2. Ballinger PW. *Merrill's Atlas of Radiographic Positions and Radiographic Procedures.* 5th Ed. St. Louis: CV Mosby, 1982, pp. 46–52.
3. Barr LL, Babcock DS. Sonography of the normal elbow. *AJR* 1991;157:793–798.
4. Beals RK. The normal carrying angle of the elbow. A radiographic study of 422 patients. *Clin Orthop* 1976;119:194–196.
5. Beltran J. The elbow. In: Beltran J, ed. *MRI: Musculoskeletal System.* 4th Ed. Philadelphia: JB Lippincott, 1990, pp. 2–11.
6. Berquist TH. The elbow and wrist. *Top Magn Reson Imag* 1989;1:15–27.
7. Blane CE, Kling TF Jr, Andrews JC, DiPietro MA, Hensinger RN. Arthrography in the posttraumatic elbow in children. *AJR* 1984;143:17–21.
8. Bledsoe RC, Izenstark JL. Displacement of fat pads in disease and injury of the elbow. *Radiology* 1959;73:717–724.
9. Bohrer SP. The fat pad sign following elbow trauma. Its usefulness and reliability in suspecting "invisible" fractures. *Clin Radiol* 1970;21:90–94.
10. Borden S IV. Roentgen recognition of acute plastic bowing of the forearm in children. *AJR* 1975;125:524–530.
11. Brody AS, Ball WS, Towbin RB. Computed arthrotomography as an adjunct to pediatric arthrography. *Radiology* 1989;170:99–102.
12. Brogdon BG, Crow NE. Little Leaguer's elbow. *AJR* 1960;83:671–675.
13. Bunnell DH, Bassett LW. The elbow. In: Bassett LW, Gold RH, Seeger LL, eds. *MRI Atlas of the Musculoskeletal System.* London: Martin Dunitz, 1989, pp. 129–138.
14. Bunnell DH, Fisher DA, Bassett LW, Gold RH, Ellman H. Elbow joint: Normal anatomy on MR images. *Radiology* 1987;165:527–531.
15. Chessare JW, Rogers LF, White H, Tachdjian MO. Injuries of the medial epicondylar ossification center of the humerus. *AJR* 1977;129:49–55.
16. Cone RO, Szabo R, Resnick D, Gelberman R, Taleisnik J, Gilula LA. Computed tomography of the normal radioulnar joints. *Invest Radiol* 1983;18:541–545.
17. D'Ambrosia R, Zink W. Fractures of the elbow in children. *Pediatr Ann* 1982;11:541–553.
18. DeHaven KE, Evarts CM. Throwing injuries of the elbow in athletes. *Orthop Clin North Am* 1973;4:801–808.
19. De Smet AA, Fisher DR, Graf BK, Lange RH. Osteochondritis dissecans of the knee: Value of MR imaging in determining lesion stability and the presence of articular cartilage defects. *AJR* 1990;155:549–553.
20. Eto RT, Anderson PW, Harley JD. Elbow arthrography with the application of tomography. *Radiology* 1975;115:283–288.
21. Firooznia H, Golimbu CN, Rafii M, Rauschning W, Weinreb JC. *MRI and CT of the Musculoskeletal System.* St. Louis: Mosby-Year Book, 1992.
22. Fowles JV, Kassab MT. Displaced supracondylar fracture of the elbow in children. *J Bone Joint Surg* 1974;56B:490–500.
23. Franklin PD, Dunlop RW, Whitelaw G, Jacques E Jr, Blickman

JG, Shapiro JH. Computed tomography of the normal and traumatized elbow. *J Comput Assist Tomogr* 1988;12:817–823.

24. Giannini S, Lipparini M, Della Villa S, Calzolari F. Ultrasonography in pathological conditions of muscles, tendons and joints. *Ital J Orthop Traumatol* 1987;13:253–259.

25. Gore RM, Rogers LF, Bowerman J, Suker J, Compere CL. Osseous manifestations of elbow stress associated with sports activities. *AJR* 1980;134:971–977.

26. Greenspan A, Norman A. Radial head-capitellum view: An expanded imaging approach to elbow injury. *Radiology* 1987;164: 272–274.

27. Greenspan A, Norman A. The radial head, capitellum view: Useful technique in elbow trauma. *AJR* 1982;138:1186–1188.

28. Greenspan A, Norman A, Rosen H. Radial head-capitellum view in elbow trauma: Clinical application and radiographic-anatomic correlation. *AJR* 1984;143:355–359.

29. Grundy A, Murphy G, Guest P, Jack L. The value of the radial head-capitellum view in radial head trauma. *Br J Radiol* 1985;58:965–967.

30. Hall-Craggs MA, Shorvon PJ, Chapman M. Assessment of the radial head-capitellum view and the dorsal fat-pad sign in acute elbow trauma. *AJR* 1985;145:607–609.

31. Hindman BW, Schreiber RR, Wiss DA, Ghilarducci MJ, Avolio RE. Supracondylar fractures of the humerus: Prediction of the cubitus varus deformity with CT. *Radiology* 1988;168:513–515.

32. Hudson TM. Elbow arthrography. *Radiol Clin North Am* 1981;19: 227–241.

33. Hudson TM. Joint fluoroscopy before arthrography: Detection and evaluation of loose bodies. *Skeletal Radiol* 1984;12:199–203.

34. Keats TE, Teeslink R, Diamond AE, Williams JH. Normal axial relationships of the major joints. *Radiology* 1966;87:904–907.

35. Koski JM. Ultrasonography of the elbow joint. *Rheumatol Int* 1990;10:91–94.

36. Lacquerriere P. De la necessite d'employer une technique radiographique speciale pour obtenir certains details squelettiques. *J Radiol Electrol* 1918;3:145–148.

37. Lindblom K. Arthrography. *J Fac Radiol* 1952;3:151–163.

38. Macrander SJ. The elbow. In: Middleton WD, Lawson TL, eds. *Anatomy and MRI of the Joints. A Multiplanar Atlas.* New York: Raven Press, 1989, pp. 49–81.

39. Magid D, Fishman EK. Imaging of musculoskeletal trauma in three dimensions. An integrated two-dimensional/three-dimensional approach with computed tomography. *Radiol Clin North Am* 1989;27:945–956.

40. McManama GB Jr, Micheli LJ, Berry MV, Sohn RS. The surgical treatment of osteochondritis of the capitellum. *Am J Sports Med* 1985;13:11–21.

41. Middleton WD, Macrander S, Kneeland JB, Froncisz W, Jesmanowicz A, Hyde JS. MR imaging of the normal elbow: Anatomic correlation. *AJR* 1987;149:543–547.

42. Miles KA, Lamont AC. Ultrasonic demonstration of the elbow fat pads. *Clin Radiol* 1989;40:602–604.

43. Milgram JW. Synovial osteochondromatosis. *J Bone Joint Surg* 1977;59A:792–801.

44. Milgram J, Rogers LF, Miller JW. Osteochondral fractures: Mechanisms of injury and fate of fragments. *AJR* 1978;130:651–658.

45. Miller GK, Drennan DB, Maylahn DJ. Treatment of displaced segmental radial-head fractures. Long-term follow-up. *J Bone Joint Surg* 1981;63A:712–717.

46. Mink JH, Eckardt JJ, Grant TT. Arthrography in recurrent dislocation of the elbow. *AJR* 1981;136:1242–1244.

47. Mitsunaga MM, Adishian DA, Bianco AJ Jr. Osteochondritis dissecans of the capitellum. *J Trauma* 1982;22:53–55.

48. Morrey BF, An K-N. Functional anatomy of the ligaments of the elbow. *Clin Orthop* 1985;201:84–90.

49. Murphy WA, Siegel MJ. Elbow fat pads with new signs and extended differential diagnosis. *Radiology* 1977;124:659–665.

50. Nelson SW. Some important diagnostic and technical fundamentals in the radiology of trauma, with particular emphasis on skeletal trauma. *Radiol Clin North Am* 1966;4:241–259.

51. Netter FH. *Atlas of Human Anatomy.* Summit, NJ: Ciba-Geigy, 1989, pp. 406–425.

52. Ozonoff MB. *Pediatric Orthopedic Radiology.* 2nd Ed. Philadelphia: WB Saunders, 1992.

53. Page AC. Critical evaluation of the radial head–capitellum view in elbow trauma. *AJR* 1986;146:81–82.

54. Patel RB, Barton P, Green L. CT of isolated elbow in evaluation of trauma: A modified technique. *Comput Radiol* 1984;8:1–4.

55. Pavlov H, Ghelman B, Warren RF. Double-contrast arthrography of the elbow. *Radiology* 1979;130:87–95.

56. Pitt MJ, Speer DP. Imaging of the elbow with an emphasis on trauma. *Radiol Clin North Am* 1990;28:293–305.

57. Rogers LF. Fractures and dislocations of the elbow. *Semin Roentgenol* 1978;13:97–107.

58. Rogers LF. Roentgenology of fractures and dislocations. In: Felson B, ed. *A Primer of Computed Tomography.* New York: Grune and Stratton, 1978, pp. 91–101.

59. Rogers LF, Malave S Jr, White H, Tachdjian MO. Plastic bowing, torus and greenstick supracondylar fractures of the humerus: Radiographic clues to obscure fractures of the elbow in children. *Radiology* 1978;128:145–150.

60. Sauser DD, Thordarson SH, Fahr LM. Imaging of the elbow. *Radiol Clin North Am* 1990;28:923–940.

61. Seltzer SE, Finberg HJ, Weissman BN. Arthrosonography: Technique, sonographic anatomy, and pathology. *Invest Radiol* 1980;15:19–28.

62. Silberstein MJ, Brodeur AE, Graviss ER, Luisiri A. Some vagaries of the medial epicondyle. *J Bone Joint Surg* 1981;63A:524–528.

63. Singson RD, Feldman F, Rosenberg ZS. Elbow joint: assessment with double-contrast CT arthrography. *Radiology* 1986;160:167–173.

64. St John JN, Palmaz JC. The cubital tunnel in ulnar entrapment neuropathy. *Radiology* 1986;158:119–123.

65. Teng MM, Murphy WA, Gilula LA, et al. Elbow arthrography: A reassessment of the technique. *Radiology* 1984;153:611–613.

66. Thompson HC III, Garcia A. Myositis ossificans: Aftermath of elbow injuries. *Clin Orthop* 1967;50:129–134.

67. Tibone JE, Stoltz M. Fractures of the radial head and neck in children. *J Bone Joint Surg* 1981;63A:100–106.

68. Torg JS, Pollack H, Sweterlitsch P. The effect of competitive pitching on the shoulders and elbows of preadolescent baseball players. *Pediatrics* 1972;49:267–272.

69. Tuckman G, Wirth CZ. Synovial osteochondromatosis of the shoulder: MR findings. *J Comput Assist Tomogr* 1989;13:360–361.

70. Turek S. *Orthopaedics.* 3rd Ed. Philadelphia: JB Lippincott, 1977, pp. 866–884.

71. Veihweger G. Zum Problem der deutung der knochernen Gebilde distal des Epikondylus medialis humeri. *Fortschr Geb Rontgenstr Nuklearmed Erganzungsbd* 1957;86:643–652.

72. Wadsworth TG. Introduction. In: Wadsworth TG, ed. *The Elbow.* New York: Churchill Livingstone, 1982, pp. 7–31.

73. Wadsworth TG. The external compression syndrome of the ulnar nerve at the cubital tunnel. *Clin Orthop* 1977;124:189–204.

74. Weissman BNW, Sledge CB. *Orthopedic Radiology.* Philadelphia: WB Saunders, 1986, pp. 173–177.

75. Williams PL, Warwick R. *Gray's Anatomy of the Human Body.* 36th British Ed. Philadelphia: WB Saunders, 1980, pp. 359–377, 571–583, 702–708, 1098–1103.

76. Woodward AH, Bianco AJ Jr. Osteochondritis dissecans of the elbow. *Clin Orthop* 1975;110:35–41.

77. Yousefzadeh DK, Jackson JH Jr. Lipohemarthrosis of the elbow joint. *Radiology* 1978;128:643–645.

Diagnostic Arthroscopy of the Elbow

Surgical Technique and Arthroscopic and Portal Anatomy

William G. Carson, Jr., M.D. *and John F. Meyers*, M.D.

Arthroscopy is most commonly used to diagnose and treat disorders of the knee. Due to technical advances in arthroscopic equipment, the development of various arthroscopic techniques for elbow arthroscopy, and the existing knowledge of arthroscopic anatomy of the elbow (both intra- and extraarticular), arthroscopy of the elbow is now possible. The value of diagnostic arthroscopy of the elbow has been well established; the visualization obtained with arthroscopy far exceeds that which may be obtained even with multiple arthrotomies about this joint.

Arthroscopy of the elbow is a technically demanding surgical procedure, and attention to detail is essential for a safe and reproducible arthroscopic examination. A thorough knowledge of the extraarticular portal anatomy of the elbow is necessary because the arthroscopic instruments must be placed through deep muscle layers and near important neurovascular structures. In addition to potential injury to nearby neurovascular structures about the elbow, other anatomic barriers exist such as a tightly constrained joint that precludes marked distention, and the fact that manipulation of the elbow does not improve visualization or advancement of the arthroscopic instruments within the elbow.

The first mention of arthroscopy of the elbow in the orthopedic literature was by Michael Burman in 1931 (4); he reported on arthroscopy performed on cadavers using a 3-mm-diameter endoscope. He stated that the el-bow was "unsuitable for examination" and that "the anterior puncture of the elbow is out of the question." In 1971, Watanabe developed the 1.7-mm #24 arthroscope for use in small joints (24). Following this development, various surgical approaches to elbow arthroscopy were described, including those of Ito (14,15) and Maeda (20), all in 1980. In 1981, Ito (16) reported a clinical study of elbow arthroscopy in the Japanese literature based on 226 cases. In 1983, Hempfling (13) described the prone position for elbow arthroscopy. In 1985, Guhl (12) reported a series of elbow arthroscopies of 45 cases. Also in 1985, Andrews and Carson (1–3,5) reported 12 cases of elbow arthroscopy and reviewed the arthroscopic technique and anatomy of the elbow. In addition to the cadaver and clinical studies described above, Lanny Johnson (18) has presented an excellent description of the technique of elbow arthroscopy and intraarticular pathology.

As elbow arthroscopy became more common, the incidence of neurovascular complications increased. In 1986, Lynch et al. (19) performed cadaver studies demonstrating the extraarticular portal anatomy and the proximity of neurovascular structures. Also in 1986, Small (22) reviewed the complications of arthroscopic surgery, including the small joints such as the elbow. Casscells (9) and Thomas et al. (23) reviewed complications of elbow arthroscopy in 1987, and Carson (6) reviewed various arthroscopic elbow complications in 1988.

INDICATIONS

Arthroscopy of the elbow is a relatively new application of arthroscopy (1–3,5–8) and at the present time is indicated for the following:

1. Extraction of loose bodies
2. Evaluation and treatment of osteochondritis dissecans of the capitellum
3. Evaluation and debridement of chondral or osteochondral lesions of the radial head
4. Debridement and lysis of adhesions of posttraumatic or certain degenerative processes about the elbow
5. Partial synovectomy in rheumatoid disease
6. Partial excision of humeral or olecranon osteophytes

Although arthroscopy of the elbow in the acute situation is less clearly indicated, it can be used to evaluate subtle fractures of the capitellum or radial head.

Use of arthroscopy for bony ankylosis and severe fibrous ankylosis is contraindicated because arthroscopic instruments cannot be introduced into the elbow. Surgical procedures such as anterior transposition of the ulnar nerve or other procedures that alter the elbow anatomy so that neurovascular structures may be jeopardized are also contraindications for elbow arthroscopy.

INSTRUMENTATION

Surgical techniques for elbow arthroscopy do not differ significantly from those used in other joints except that greater care must be taken to avoid scuffing or gouging the articular cartilage of the distal humerus, radial head, or olecranon. The elbow joint is inherently stable, and there is little room in which to maneuver the various instruments. Elbow arthroscopy should be performed slowly and deliberately to avoid slipping out of the elbow capsule, creating multiple entries of the various cannulas into the joint (5).

Hand-held instruments such as basket forceps, grasping forceps, rongeurs, punches, and probes are commonly used for elbow arthroscopy. Motorized instruments used include synovial resectors, trimmers, cutters, etc. The use of motorized instruments is safer because repeated passes are avoided. Repeated passes can create multiple capsular holes and increase the extravasation of fluid about the elbow, increasing the risk of damage to nearby neurovascular structures. Whether hand-held or motorized, all instruments should be used carefully within the elbow. The instruments should not be wedged between articular cartilage surfaces due to the possibility of damaging the articular cartilage. As with any arthroscopic surgery, the instruments should always be kept in full view.

The arthroscopic systems used on the larger joints are also used on the elbow. A 4-mm, 30° angled arthroscope provides optimal visualization of the elbow. Smaller arthroscopes may be used to prevent cartilage damage. "Small joint system" arthroscopic equipment is helpful in visualizing smaller spaces within the elbow joint; however, the overall field of view is somewhat narrower in small joint systems.

ANESTHESIA

General anesthesia is commonly used for elbow arthroscopy because it affords complete comfort and provides total muscle relaxation. Intrascalene or axillary blocks can also be used; however, some practitioners feel their use requires considerable expertise and increases the difficulty of immediate postoperative neurovascular evaluation. Ito (17) has advocated the use of local anesthesia for diagnostic arthroscopy. Minkoff (personal communication) advocates local anesthesia for diagnostic and surgical elbow arthroscopy because the patient may communicate with the operating surgeon when instruments are placed in proximity to the nerves about the elbow. Intravenous regional anesthesia may also be used; however, the use of dual tourniquets about the upper arm may compromise elbow exposure and cause vascular engorgement and edema, thus compromising visualization of the joint.

SURGICAL TECHNIQUE

We routinely use a properly padded tourniquet placed as high on the upper arm and as near the axilla as possible. When using a tourniquet control, care should be taken to use an appropriately sized cuff and to limit tourniquet use to no more than 2 hours (21).

The patient is placed in the supine position with the upper arm and forearm hanging free over the edge of the operating table. The hand and forearm are placed in a prefabricated forearm and wrist gauntlet connected to an overhead suspension device so that the elbow is flexed to 90° (Fig. 1). Traction is applied to the arm through a pulley and weight system, suspending the arm and keeping the elbow flexed at 90°. This position provides excellent access to both the medial and lateral aspects of the elbow. The forearm may be freely pronated and supinated throughout the surgical procedure. The elbow must remain in this 90° flexed position at all times when examining the anterior structures of the elbow arthroscopically to maintain complete relaxation of the neurovascular structures in the antecubital fossa (1,5–8).

Extremity drapes are used to drape the upper arm and the patient. A sterile transparent plastic drape is used to cover the forearm gauntlet. The surgeon sits on the radial side of the patient with the first assistant on the axilla side of the elbow. A Mayo stand can be placed at the end of the table, and the second assistant or scrub technician may stand behind the Mayo stand. Video equipment is placed opposite the patient.

Some surgeons have proposed placing the patient in a prone position (13; and Whipple, Poehling, and Sisco, personal communications). The prone position provides ready access to both the anterior and posterior aspects of the elbow and allows gravity to help displace the neurovascular structures in the antecubital fossa away from the entering instruments. When used in conjunction with the proximal medial portal, this position improves mobility of the instruments within the joint and provides an improved view of the anterior joint (Fig. 2).

After anesthesia has been administered and the patient's position is stabilized, the bony anatomic landmarks are outlined with a marking pen prior to initiation of the procedure. Since large amounts of extravasation of fluid are present during the arthroscopic procedures, marking the landmarks facilitates their identification during surgery. The landmarks that are marked include the radial head and the lateral humeral epicondyle on the lateral side of the elbow, and the medial humeral epicondyle on the medial aspect of the elbow (Fig. 3). The olecranon is identified posteriorly.

PORTALS

The most commonly used portals in elbow arthroscopy are the anterolateral, anteromedial, and posterolateral. Other portals have been described for elbow arthroscopy (11,14–16,18,20,24), including several lateral portals (12) and the anteromedial supracondylar or proximal medial portal (17). The majority of arthro-

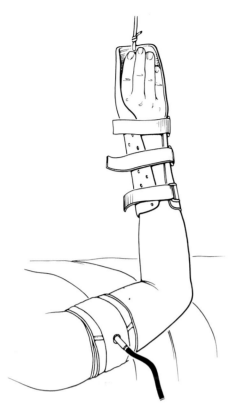

FIG. 1. The hand and forearm are placed in a prefabricated forearm and wrist gauntlet, which is connected to an overhead suspension device so that the elbow is flexed to 90°.

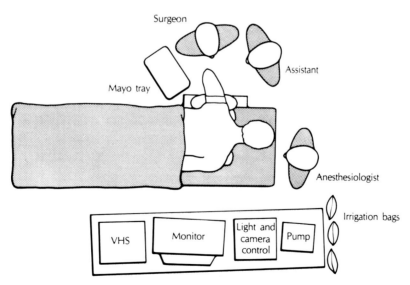

FIG. 2. Operating room setup for arthroscopy of the elbow, with patient in prone position.

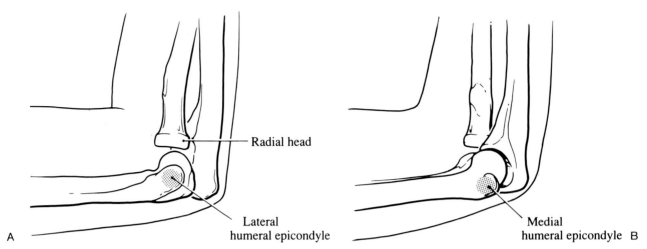

FIG. 3. Bony landmarks. **A:** Radial head and lateral humeral epicondyle on the lateral aspect of the elbow. **B:** Medial humeral epicondyle on the medial aspect of the elbow.

scopic surgical procedures performed on the elbow use a combination of the anterolateral, anteromedial, and posterolateral portals. Two accessory portals, the direct lateral portal and the direct posterior portal, can be added if required. The proximal medial portal may be used as a primary diagnostic portal.

Prior to the insertion of the arthroscope into a portal, the elbow should be maximally distended with saline using a 50-cc syringe connected to intravenous tubing and an 18-gauge spinal needle. The most reliable insertion site for this needle is through the triangular area over the lateral aspect of the elbow, which is bordered by the radial head, the lateral humeral epicondyle, and the tip of the olecranon (Fig. 4). This area is often used to aspirate the elbow for hemarthrosis. When penetrating this area, the 18-gauge needle traverses skin, a thin subcutaneous

layer, the anconeus muscle, and the capsule. Proper placement into the elbow joint is verified by brisk backflow from the needle. After entry into the joint is verified, the needle is removed, and the elbow is left maximally distended. At this point the primary diagnostic arthroscopic portal may be established.

Anterolateral Portal

The anterolateral portal is the standard diagnostic portal for elbow arthroscopy and is usually the first arthroscopic portal established. After the elbow is flexed at 90° and maximally distended, the 18-gauge spinal needle is placed 3 cm distal and 2 cm anterior to the lateral humeral epicondyle (Fig. 5) and aimed toward the center of

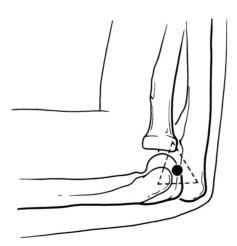

FIG. 4. Insertion site for the 18-gauge spinal needle for initial distention of the elbow is located through the triangular area bordered by the lateral humeral epicondyle, the radial head, and the tip of the olecranon.

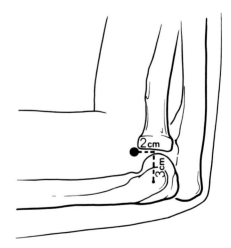

FIG. 5. The anterolateral portal is located approximately 3 cm distal and 2 cm anterior to the lateral humeral epicondyle.

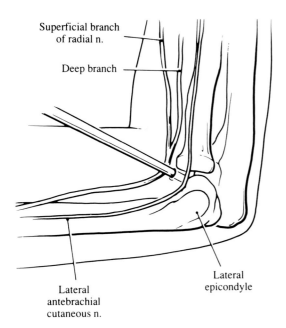

FIG. 6. The arthroscope courses just anterior to the radial head to visualize the anterior structures of the elbow joint.

the joint. The course of the needle lies just anterior to the radial head, which can be identified by pronating and supinating the forearm. Entry into the elbow joint is confirmed by free backflow of the fluid previously placed into the elbow.

Once proper placement of the 18-gauge needle is confirmed and the elbow is maximally distended, the larger arthroscopic instruments, such as the arthroscope itself and the cannula system, can be introduced (Fig. 6). The cannula system is introduced by making a small incision in the skin, taking care to avoid injury to the underlying subcutaneous nerves. Close attention should be given to the subcutaneous nerves about the elbow when establishing elbow portals. The #11 blade is laid against the skin, and the skin is then pulled across the blade. This incision and underlying subcutaneous tissues may then be deepened using a hemostat (19). The lateral and posterior antebrachial cutaneous nerves must be avoided. The lateral antebrachial cutaneous nerve is the terminal branch of the musculocutaneous nerve and pierces the brachial fascia just lateral to the biceps tendon just proximal to the elbow joint. It then divides into an anterior and posterior branch, with the anterior branch supplying the skin over the anterolateral portion of the forearm. The

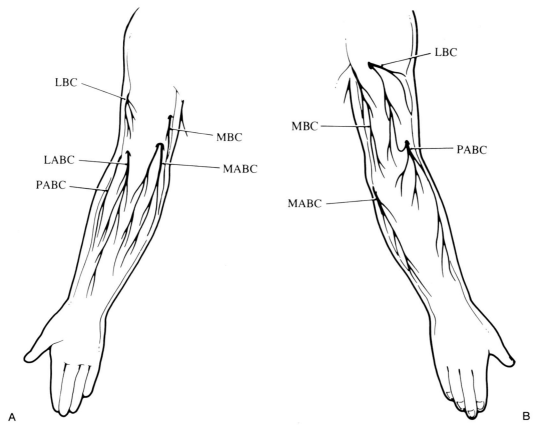

FIG. 7. A: Anatomy of the lateral antebrachial cutaneous nerve (LABC). **B:** Anatomy of the posterior antebrachial cutaneous nerve (PABC). LBC, lateral brachial cutaneous; MBC, medial brachial cutaneous; MABC, medial antebrachial cutaneous.

posterior branch passes over the lateral humeral epicondyle and supplies the skin of the radial border of the forearm (Fig. 7A). The posterior antebrachial cutaneous nerve is a branch of the radial nerve and pierces the brachial fascia in the lower two-thirds of the arm, supplying the skin behind the lateral humeral epicondyle and dorsal aspect of the forearm (Fig. 7B).

At this point a blunt trocar is used because it can be readily inserted through the subcutaneous fat and the muscles. Using the blunt trocar when inserting the cannulas minimizes damage to nearby neurovascular structures and articular cartilage. Once resistance is noted, the sharp trocar can be inserted through the deeper fascial and capsular layers. The blunt trocar is then reintroduced to enter the elbow joint itself.

When inserting the trocar and cannula system, great care must be given to the angle of insertion. The instruments should be directed toward the center of the elbow with the elbow flexed at 90° at all times. Once the capsule is entered, free backflow of fluid will be noted through the cannula, verifying entrance into the joint. At this time the arthroscope is inserted and diagnostic arthroscopy is begun.

Continuous distention of the elbow is maintained using two 3-liter bags of normal saline elevated above the patient and attached to the arthroscope, thereby allowing gravity distention to distend the elbow. If additional inflow is required, a 50-cc syringe connected to the arthroscopic cannula may be used to provide further distention manually. Infusion pumps also provide excellent distention of the elbow. Distention may also be maintained with a blood transfusion cuff pump, keeping the pressure at approximately 30 mm Hg (21).

When a second arthroscopic portal is established (as described below), a separate cannula may be inserted for distention and improved visualization. Suction may be intermittently placed on the arthroscopic sleeve to remove any cloudy fluid or debris. Unless cleansing is required, the sleeve is usually left clamped off to maintain distention pressure within the elbow.

Anterolateral Portal Anatomy

During the establishment of the anterolateral portal, the arthroscope passes anterior to the radial head, through the extensor carpi radialis brevis muscle, and then through the lateral capsule before entering the joint (1,19) (Fig. 8). The arthroscope may pass from 4 mm (19) to 7 mm (1) beneath the radial nerve when establishing the anterolateral portal. The radial nerve is located between the brachialis and brachioradialis over the distal aspect of the arm. As the nerve passes in front of the lateral humeral epicondyle, it divides into a superficial branch, which runs on the deep side of the brachioradialis, and a deep motor branch, which pierces the supinator muscle to supply the extensor muscles of the forearm (Fig. 9). Lynch et al. (19) have demonstrated that the arthroscopic instruments pass within a mean distance of 4 mm of the radial nerve, regardless of the flexion or extension of the elbow, when the elbow is not distended with fluid. However, when 35 to 40 cc of fluid was inserted into the elbow capsule, the radial nerve moved an additional 7 mm anteriorly (19). Thus maximum distention of the elbow should be maintained at all times, particularly when establishing the initial arthroscopic portals.

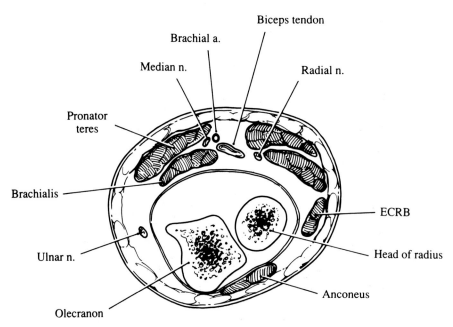

FIG. 8. Cross-sectional view of elbow at level of anterolateral and anteromedial portals with joint distention. ECRB, extensor carpi radialis brevis muscle.

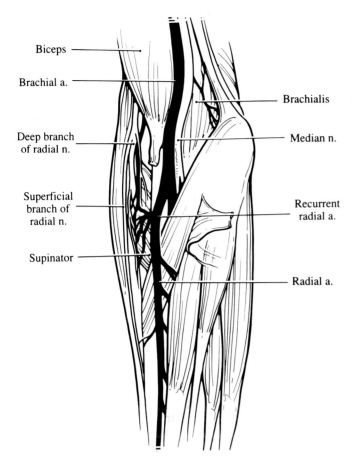

FIG. 9. Neurovascular structures of antecubital fossa of the elbow.

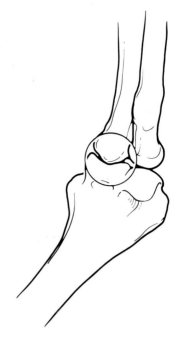

FIG. 10. Intraarticular structures that can be visualized from the anterolateral portal are the distal humerus and trochlear ridges and the coronoid process of the ulna.

Arthroscopic Anatomy of Anterolateral Portal

Intraarticular structures of the elbow that can be seen from the anterolateral portal are the distal humerus, trochlear ridges, and coronoid process of the ulna (Fig. 10). Flexion and extension of the elbow allows the arthroscopist to see the coronoid process of the ulna; extending the elbow provides a better view of the medial and lateral trochlear ridges and the trochlear notch of the distal humerus. By slowly retracting and angling the 30° arthroscope toward the radial head, the medial aspect of the radial head and superior articulation between the ulna and radial head can be partially seen.

Anteromedial Portal

After the anterolateral portal has been entered, the anteromedial portal can be safely established by direct intraarticular visualization. At times a 3.5-mm synovial whisker may be needed to increase visualization when establishing the second arthroscopic portal or when secondary instrumentation is performed in the elbow. A synovectomy of the villi appears to be safe and does not

violate the elbow capsule. Once proper visualization is obtained through the anterolateral portal, the anteromedial portal is identified approximately 2 cm anterior and 2 cm distal to the medial humeral epicondyle (Fig. 11).

With the arthroscope in the anterolateral portal, an 18-gauge spinal needle is inserted at the entry point described above with the elbow flexed 90° and maximally distended with fluid. The needle is aimed directly toward

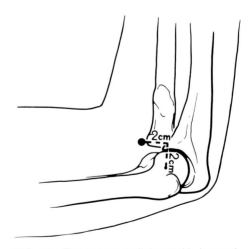

FIG. 11. The anteromedial portal is located approximately 2 cm anterior and 2 cm distal to the medial humeral epicondyle.

the center of the joint. Confirmation of the needle's entry into the joint is provided by direct visualization through the arthroscope in the anterolateral portal. The needle passes just anterior to the medial humeral epicondyle and inferior to the antecubital structures (Fig. 12).

A small incision is made in the skin, and the arthroscopic cannula and trocar system are introduced. An interchangeable cannula system is used to change freely from the anterolateral to the anteromedial portals with the various instruments. If a simple diagnostic arthroscopy is being performed, an inflow cannula can be placed through the anteromedial portal to provide better distention and visualization (Fig. 13). Because maximum distention of the elbow is being maintained at all times, the extracapsular extravasation of fluid should be monitored closely, particularly if a large inflow cannula is being used as a separate inflow system. Extracapsular extravasation is most often seen when repeated attempts have been made to establish the arthroscopic portals, resulting in multiple holes in the capsule and fluid leakage. When using an inflow cannula as a separate portal for distention, the cannula should not have any "side vents" because if the inflow cannula slips back somewhat during the arthroscopic procedure fluid will leak directly into the subcutaneous tissues (Fig. 14).

Most arthroscopic surgical procedures in the elbow are performed for pathologic processes located over the lateral aspect of the elbow, such as loose bodies or osteo-

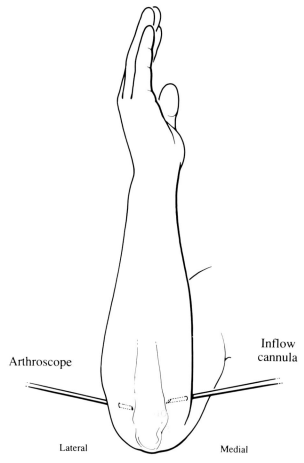

FIG. 13. Utilization of a separate inflow cannula through the anteromedial portal to obtain distention of the elbow with the arthroscope in place through the anterolateral portal.

chondritis dissecans of the capitellum. The anteromedial portal provides excellent visualization of these structures, compared with the anterolateral portal; therefore technical proficiency at establishing both portals is necessary.

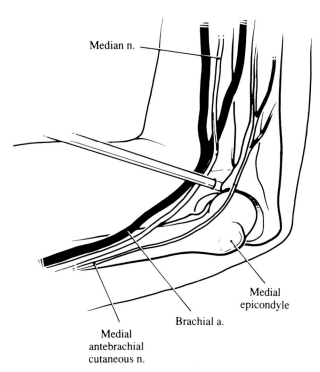

FIG. 12. The arthroscope passes just anterior to the medial humeral epicondyle to view the anterior structures of the elbow joint.

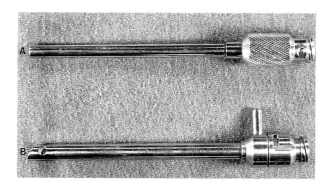

FIG. 14. Correct (**A**) and incorrect (**B**) types of inflow cannulas for distention in elbow arthroscopy.

Anteromedial Portal Anatomy

When establishing the anteromedial portal, the medial antebrachial cutaneous nerve should be avoided. This nerve divides into an anterior branch supplying the forearm and a smaller ulnar branch which courses over the medial humeral epicondyle.

In establishing the anteromedial portal, the arthroscope enters through the tendinous portion of the pronator teres and penetrates the radial aspect of the flexor digitorum superficialis and medial capsule (1). As these muscles are penetrated, the median nerve is 1 cm lateral to the arthroscope, and the brachial artery is just lateral to the median nerve. The brachial artery divides into the radial and ulnar arteries opposite the neck of the radius. The median nerve crosses the elbow joint in the antecubital fossa and passes beneath the bicipital aponeurosis and between the two heads of the pronator teres. As the arthroscope passes deeper and closer to the joint capsule, it passes within 6 mm of the median nerve and brachial artery in a nondistended elbow. When 35 to 40 cc of fluid is injected within the elbow, the median nerve and brachial artery are displaced 10 and 8 mm anteriorly, respectively, from the entering arthroscopic instruments (19). Thus it becomes readily apparent that maximum distention and 90° of flexion of the elbow is necessary to provide a safe entry for instrumentation from the medial aspect of the elbow.

Anteromedial Portal Arthroscopic Anatomy

The capitellum and radial head are best seen from the anteromedial portal. Examination of the radial head is facilitated by pronating and supinating the forearm (Fig. 15). Approximately three-fourths of the radial head can be seen utilizing this technique. At times the annular ligament may be seen coursing across the radial neck. By slowly retracting the arthroscope and directing it toward the ulna, the coronoid process is also visible. Flexion and extension of the elbow allows visualization of most of the anterior surface of the capitellum.

Posterolateral Portal

The entry point for the posterolateral portal is approximately 3 cm proximal to the olecranon tip, just superior and posterior to the lateral humeral epicondyle near the lateral border of the triceps muscle (Fig. 16). This portal is established with the elbow in 20° to 30° of flexion. The 18-gauge spinal needle is directed toward the olecranon fossa. If the joint has already been distended with fluid from the anteromedial or anterolateral portals, a capsular bulge can often be felt over the posterolateral elbow and used to identify the insertion site for the needle. Whereas the anteromedial and anterolateral portals are

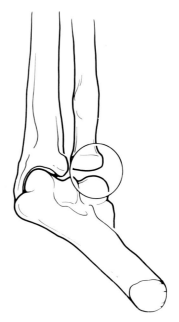

FIG. 15. The capitellum and radial head are best seen from the anteromedial portal. Examination of the radial head is facilitated by pronating and supinating the forearm.

primarily used to view the anterior aspects of the elbow, the posterolateral portal is used to complete the full evaluation of the joint, since loose bodies or osteophytes may be located in the olecranon fossa and the posterior aspect of the capitellum.

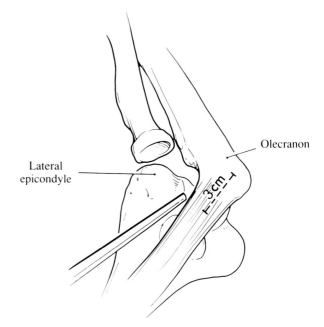

FIG. 16. The posterolateral portal is located approximately 3 cm proximal to the olecranon tip just superior and posterior to the lateral humeral epicondyle off of the lateral border of the triceps muscle.

Posterolateral Portal Anatomy

The posterior antebrachial cutaneous nerve, which courses over the posterolateral distal humerus, and the lateral brachial cutaneous nerve, which is the terminal branch of the axillary nerve, are to be avoided when establishing this portal. The trocar pierces the triceps musculature and then the posterolateral elbow capsule, and care must be taken to avoid the ulnar nerve, which lies approximately 2.5 cm medial to the center of the elbow joint.

Arthroscopic Anatomy of Posterolateral Portal

Structures that may be seen from this portal are the olecranon fossa, located over the posterior aspect of the distal humerus, and the tip of the olecranon (Fig. 17). Flexion and extension of the elbow will help delineate various portions of the distal humerus.

Proximal Medial Portal

The proximal medial portal (or supracondylar anteromedial portal) has been advocated as the primary diagnostic arthroscopic portal by Poehling (personal communication). When using this portal the patient is placed in the prone position (Fig. 2) with the shoulder and proximal arm elevated on a sandbag, which is placed on an arm board adjacent to the operating table. The usual bony landmarks are outlined with a marking pen, in-

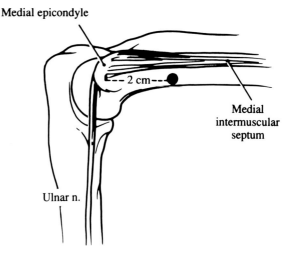

FIG. 18. Insertion site for the proximal medial portal is located 2 cm proximal to the medial humeral epicondyle anterior to the palpable medial intermuscular septum.

cluding the medial and lateral humeral epicondyle, the medial intermuscular septum, the radial head, and the olecranon. The joint is distended with 35 to 40 cc of fluid injected into the elbow laterally through the "soft spot" bordered by the radial head, olecranon, and lateral humeral epicondyle. The proximal medial portal is located 2 cm proximal to the medial humeral epicondyle (Fig. 18). Injury to the ulnar nerve may be avoided by remaining anterior to the easily palpated intermuscular septum. A small incision in the skin is made with the tip of a #11 scalpel blade. The cannula and blunt trocar are then inserted, staying anterior to the intermuscular septum and in contact with the anterior humerus. The trocar is directed toward the radial head during insertion. The elbow capsule is then punctured, and the arthroscope is entered. Because the arthroscope is entering more proximal than in the anteromedial or anterolateral portals, the overall view of the anterior aspects of the elbow is increased (Fig. 19).

Accessory Portals

When pathology is encountered that is not amenable to the arthroscopic portals mentioned above, two accessory portals, the straight lateral portal and the straight posterior portal, may be used.

The straight lateral portal is located in the triangular area bordered by the lateral humeral epicondyle, the radial head, and the olecranon. Through this portal, the trocar system passes through the anconeus muscle and the posterior capsule, the same area in which the 18-gauge spinal needle is inserted for initial distention of the elbow joint. This portal may be established directly using an 18-gauge spinal needle and the sharp and blunt trocar system, or it may be made under direct visualization us-

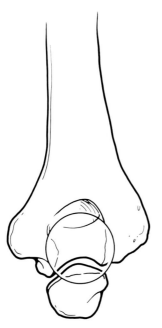

FIG. 17. Structures that may be visualized from the posterolateral portal include the olecranon fossa and the tip of the olecranon.

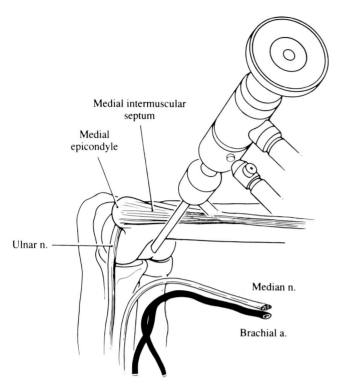

FIG. 19. Arthroscopic view of anterior aspect of the elbow utilizing the proximal medial portal.

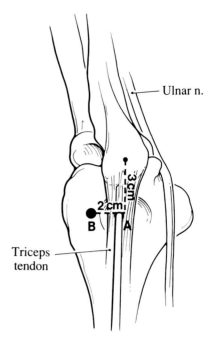

FIG. 21. The accessory posterior portal (A) is located 2 cm medial to the standard posterolateral portal (B) and passes directly through the triceps tendon.

ing the anteromedial or anterolateral portal to watch the instruments as they enter the elbow joint. When establishing this portal, the posterior antebrachial cutaneous nerve should be avoided.

The radial ulnar joint and the inferior surface of the radial head can be seen through the straight lateral portal. In addition, the undersurface of the capitellum can be followed posteriorly. At times the arthroscope will slip directly into the posterior compartment, providing a view of this area as well (Fig. 20).

The straight posterior portal is located approximately

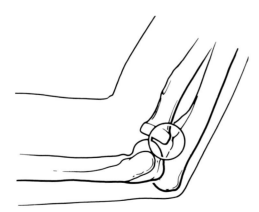

FIG. 20. Structures visualized through the straight lateral portal include the radial ulna joint and the inferior surface of the radial head.

2 cm medial to the posterolateral portal and directly traverses the triceps tendon (Fig. 21). The elbow is flexed 20° to 30° to facilitate introduction of the instruments into the joint. The straight posterior portal is useful for removing loose bodies from the posterior aspect of the elbow as well as for the occasional resection of an impinging olecranon osteophyte (3).

POSTOPERATIVE ROUTINE

At the completion of the procedure, thorough irrigation of the joint can greatly improve the patient's postoperative recovery. Irrigation is particularly important when performing debridement of adhesions or articular surfaces. This step is often neglected due to the belief that the joint has been sufficiently irrigated during the operative procedure. However, the elbow cannot be flexed and extended completely with all of the instruments in place. Thus, at the end of the surgical procedure, one inflow cannula is left in place, and the elbow is completely flexed and extended several times, alternating irrigation and suction to remove any debris thoroughly.

The arthroscopic portals may be closed with suture material or left open, depending on the preference of the surgeon and the amount of subcutaneous swelling. Local anesthetics may leak out of the capsular holes and cause a temporary nerve block, interfering with the immediate postoperative neurovascular assessment. Soft dressings are applied to the elbow, and in most cases immobilization is not required. Active range of motion of the elbow is initiated as soon as pain and swelling permit. Flexibility and strengthening exercises are usually initiated after pain and swelling are reduced and the patient's preoperative range of motion has been regained.

COMPLICATIONS

Complications of elbow arthroscopy are similar to those encountered with any arthroscopic procedure, such as infection, problems associated with the use of a tourniquet, instrument breakage, iatrogenic scuffing of articular surfaces, and neurovascular complications. Infection is infrequent with elbow arthroscopy because of the large amount of fluid passed through the joint during the surgical procedure as well as the small incisions required for the arthroscopic instrumentation.

Neurovascular complications, however, appear to be more of a problem. In a series of 21 elbow arthroscopies, Lynch et al. (19) reported one transient low radial nerve palsy, a transient low median nerve palsy, and formation of a neuroma of the medial antebrachial cutaneous nerve. It was felt that the transient low radial nerve palsy was due to overdistention of the joint, and the condition resolved in 8 hours. The transient low median nerve palsy was felt to be secondary to use of a local anesthetic. The neuroma formation of the medial antebrachial cutaneous nerve ultimately required resection.

Casscells (9) described a case of irreparable damage to the ulnar nerve during abrasion arthroplasty of the elbow. Thomas et al. (23) described a radial nerve injury during elbow arthroscopy. In a series of 45 patients, Guhl (12) reported that one patient suffered an injury to the sensory branch of the radial nerve. In a series of 24 arthroscopies reported by Andrews and Carson (1), one patient experienced a transient median nerve palsy. This transient nerve palsy was felt to be secondary to leakage of local anesthetic from the capsule, causing a temporary nerve block.

In a survey of members of the Arthroscopy Association of North America (10), 395,566 surgical arthroscopic procedures were evaluated, of which 5069 were elbow arthroscopies. The respondents were performing an average of 0.74 elbow arthroscopy per month and had been performing surgical elbow arthroscopy for an average of 3.9 years. Of this entire group, only one reported a neurovascular complication, a radial nerve injury (22).

A more common problem experienced during elbow arthroscopy appears to be postoperative paresthesias and dysesthesias. These problems could be related to the use of a tourniquet or could be due to fluid extravasation during the surgical procedure. The other consideration is actual injury as a result of traction or blunt trauma to the subcutaneous nerves around the elbow joint.

Arthroscopy of the elbow is a technically demanding surgical procedure, and significant attention to detail is essential in order to perform a safe and reproducible arthroscopic examination. Complications may be avoided by adhering to a strict surgical technique.

REFERENCES

1. Andrews JR, Carson WG. Arthroscopy of the elbow. *Arthroscopy* 1985;1:97–107.
2. Andrews JR, Carson WG. Arthroscopy of the elbow. In: McGinty JB, ed. *Techniques in Orthopaedics: Arthroscopic Surgery Update.* Rockville, MD: Aspen, 1985, pp. 183–190.
3. Andrews JR, St. Pierre RK, Carson WG. Arthroscopy of the elbow. *Clin Sports Med* 1986;5:653–662.
4. Burman MS. Arthroscopy or the direct visualization of joints. *J Bone Joint Surg* 1931;13:669–695.
5. Carson WG, Andrews JR. Arthroscopy of the elbow. In: Zarins B, Andrews J, Carson WG, eds. *Injuries to the Throwing Arm.* Philadelphia: WB Saunders, 1985, pp. 221–227.
6. Carson WG. Arthroscopy of the elbow. In: Bassett F, ed. *AAOS Instructional Course Lecture.* Vol. 37. Chicago: American Academy of Orthopaedic Surgeons, 1988, pp. 195–201.
7. Carson WG. Complications of elbow arthroscopy. In: Minkoff J, Sherman O, eds. *Arthroscopic Surgery.* Baltimore: Williams and Wilkins, 1988.
8. Carson WG. Arthroscopy of the elbow. In: Torg J, Welsh RP, eds. *Current Therapy in Sports Medicine.* Philadelphia: B.C. Decker, 1988.
9. Casscells SW. Neurovascular anatomy and elbow arthroscopy: Inherent risks [Editors comment]. *Arthroscopy* 1987;2:190.
10. DeLee JC. Complications of arthroscopy and arthroscopic surgery: Results of a national survey. *Arthroscopy* 1985;1:214–220.
11. Eriksson E, Denti M. Diagnostic and operative arthroscopy of the shoulder and elbow joint. *Ital J Sports Traumatol* 1985;7:165–188.
12. Guhl JF. Arthroscopy and arthroscopic surgery of the elbow. *Orthopaedics* 1985;8(1):290–296.
13. Hempfling H. Die endoskopische Untersuching des Ellenbogengelenkes vom dorso-radialen Zugang. *Z Orthop* 1983;121:331.
14. Ito K. The arthroscopic anatomy of the elbow joint. [In Japanese.] *Arthroscopy* 1979;4:2–9.
15. Ito K. Arthroscopy of the elbow joint—a cadaver study. [In Japanese.] *Arthroscopy* 1980;5:9–22.
16. Ito K. Arthroscopy of the elbow joint. *Arthroscopy* 1981;6:15–24.
17. Ito K. Arthroscopy of the elbow joint. In: Watanabe M, ed. *Arthroscopy of Small Joints.* New York: Igaku-Shoin, 1985, pp. 57–84.
18. Johnson LL. Elbow arthroscopy. In: *Arthroscopic Surgery: Principles and Practice.* St. Louis: C.V. Mosby, 1986, pp. 1446–1477.
19. Lynch GJ, Meyers JF, Whipple TL, Caspari RB. Neurovascular anatomy and elbow arthroscopy: Inherent risks. *Arthroscopy* 1986;2:191–197.
20. Maeda Y. Arthroscopy of the elbow joint. [In Japanese.] *Arthroscopy* 1980;5:5–8.
21. Schonholtz GJ. *Arthroscopic Surgery of the Shoulder, Elbow and Ankle.* Springfield, IL: CC Thomas, 1986, pp. 73–78.
22. Small NC. Complications in arthroscopy: On knee and other joints. *Arthroscopy* 1986;2:253–258.
23. Thomas MA, Fast A, Shapiro D. Radial nerve damage as a complication of elbow arthroscopy. *Clin Orthop* 1987;215:130–131.
24. Watanabe M. Arthroscopy of small joints. [In Japanese.] *J Jpn Orthop Assoc* 1971;45:908.

Arthroscopic Surgical Treatment
of Elbow Pathology

James R. Andrews, M.D., *and Patrick J. McKenzie*, M.D.

Arthroscopic surgery of the elbow has undergone growth and development in recent years similar to that of knee and shoulder arthroscopy. Since the first description of diagnostic arthroscopy of the elbow by Watanabe, both diagnostic and operative procedures have been more thoroughly defined. As with the knee and shoulder, the elbow joint is readily accessible to arthroscopic evaluation. However, penetration of the deep muscular layers and the close proximity of the major neurovascular structures about the elbow make elbow arthroscopy more technically demanding than arthroscopy of the knee and shoulder.

The first and most readily apparent advantage of elbow arthroscopy over open surgical procedures is that arthroscopy requires only small puncture holes through the tissue and capsule surrounding the elbow joint. By avoiding a large capsular incision, many of the problems of postoperative scarring and capsular contraction of the elbow can be avoided. Second, the small arthroscopic surgical portals allow a much more aggressive postoperative physical therapy regimen without the concern for wound healing required with an open procedure. Third, by using anteromedial, anterolateral, straight lateral, and posterolateral portals, a much more thorough visual inspection of the entire elbow joint is possible than through an arthrotomy incision. Finally, arthroscopic surgical procedures of the elbow have a much reduced risk of intraarticular infection compared with an open arthrotomy procedure.

The disadvantages of elbow arthroscopy are related to the surgical procedure itself. The failure to adhere to strict anatomic and technical guidelines may lead to

damage of the major neurovascular structures about the elbow. In addition, arthroscopy may require slightly more operative time compared with an open arthrotomy because of its more demanding technical requirements.

At the present time, elbow arthroscopy is used for (a) diagnosis of patients with chronic elbow pain of undetermined etiology; (b) loose body removal; (c) evaluation and debridement of osteochondritic lesions of the capitellum; (d) excision of osteophytes, especially off the posterior and posteromedial tip of the olecranon; (e) synovectomy for systemic inflammatory conditions such as rheumatoid arthritis; and (f) lysis and debridement of posttraumatic and postsurgical adhesions. The use of elbow arthroscopy in the acute setting, such as evaluation of fractures of the capitellum, radial head, or olecranon, has not been as clearly defined (1).

Contraindications to elbow arthroscopy include (a) severe bony fibrous ankylosis that prevents introduction of the arthroscope into the elbow; (b) bleeding disorders that have not been corrected medically; (c) concurrent infection; (d) previous surgical procedures (i.e., anterior transposition of the ulnar nerve) that alter the neurovascular anatomy around the elbow such that placement of the usual arthroscopic portals could produce neurovascular injury (3).

ARTHROSCOPIC SURGICAL APPROACH
TO THE ELBOW

The basic anatomic and technical considerations for performing elbow arthroscopy have been well described

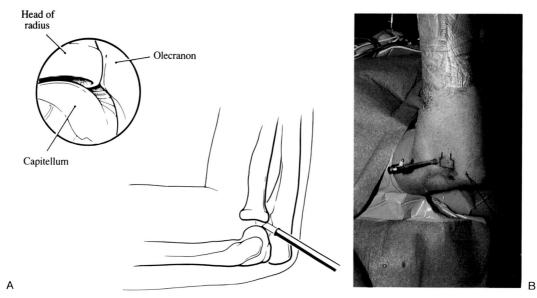

FIG. 1. A, B: Anterior lateral portal.

in the preceding chapter, and these will not be reviewed at this time. Our initial approach for arthroscopic surgical procedures of the elbow is the establishment of an anterolateral portal, through which the anterior aspect of the elbow, and more specifically the anterior capsule, coronoid process, and trochlea can be well visualized (Fig. 1). Next, an anteromedial portal can be established under direct visualization, and the remainder of the anterior capsule, radial head, and capitellum can be visualized (Fig. 2). After the anterior aspect of the elbow is evaluated, a straight lateral portal is established, through which the capitellum, radial head, and lateral aspect of the olecranon can be well visualized (Fig. 3). After a thor-

ough evaluation of these structures, a posterolateral portal may be established under direct visualization. The posterior, posteromedial, and posterolateral tip of the olecranon and the olecranon fossa can be thoroughly examined through this portal (Fig. 4). The remainder of the posterior aspect of the elbow can also be seen through the posterolateral portal.

Arthroscopic surgical procedures of the anterior aspect of the elbow require both anterolateral and anteromedial portals. Depending on the pathology, the arthroscope may be introduced through either the anterolateral or anteromedial portal. The arthroscopic surgical instruments are then introduced through the opposite portal

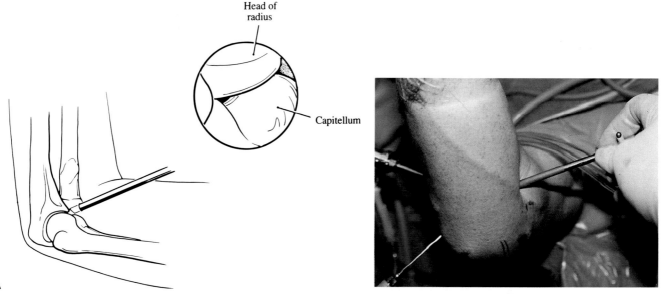

FIG. 2. A, B: Anterior medial portal.

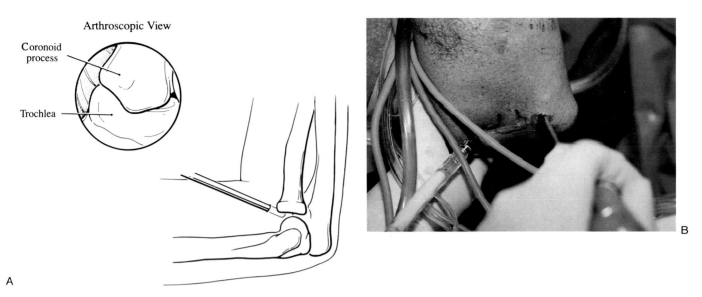

FIG. 3. A, B: Straight lateral portal.

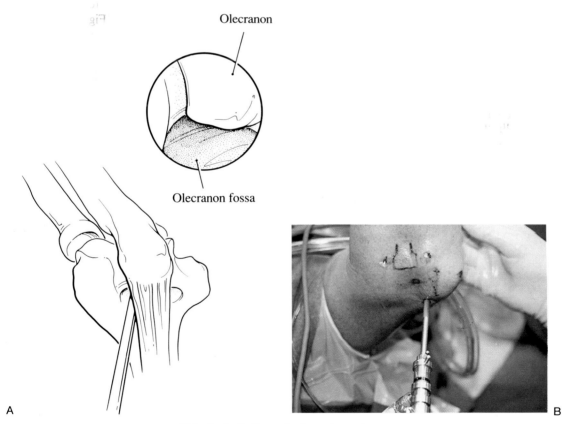

FIG. 4. A, B: Posterior lateral portal.

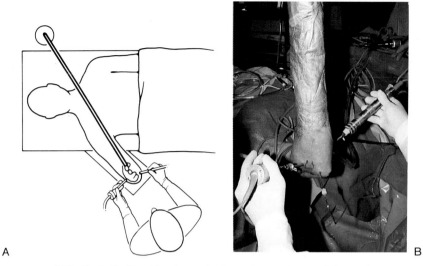

FIG. 5. A, B: Combined anterior lateral–anterior medial portal.

(Fig. 5). In addressing lesions on the lateral side of the elbow, the arthroscope and the arthroscopic surgical instruments are brought through separate stab incisions in the "soft spot" on the lateral side of the elbow (Fig. 6). In addressing posterior lesions of the olecranon, posteromedial olecranon, and olecranon fossa, the arthroscope is introduced through the posterolateral portal, and the operative instruments are brought through a straight posterior portal through the triceps tendon (Fig. 7).

At the completion of any arthroscopic surgical procedure on the elbow, a Hemovac drain is left in the elbow joint through one of the arthroscopic portals. The elbow is then dressed in a sterile bulky dressing that allows frequent neurovascular checks of the extremity postoperatively. This dressing is changed and the drains are pulled on the first postoperative day so that physical therapy may be initiated (2).

ARTHROSCOPIC SURGICAL TREATMENT OF SPECIFIC LESIONS

Loose Bodies

Removal of loose bodies has become one of the most common indications for elbow arthroscopy. Loose bodies within the elbow may be composed of osteocartilaginous tissue, cartilaginous tissue, or fibrous tissue. The osteocartilaginous loose bodies are most often the result of osteochondritic lesions of the capitellum, osteochondral fractures from lateral compression injuries, and synovial diseases such as synovial chondromotosis. Cartilaginous loose bodies are usually the result of traumatic shearing off of the articular cartilage surface, with the resulting free fragment of cartilage becoming a loose body. Fibrous loose bodies are usually the result of hypertrophied

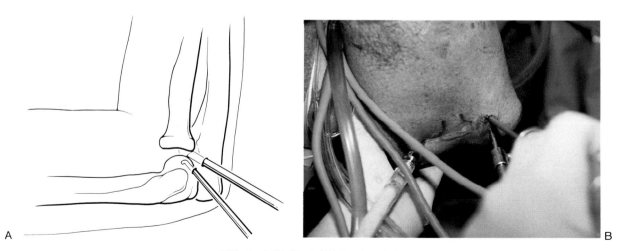

FIG. 6. A, B: Straight lateral portal.

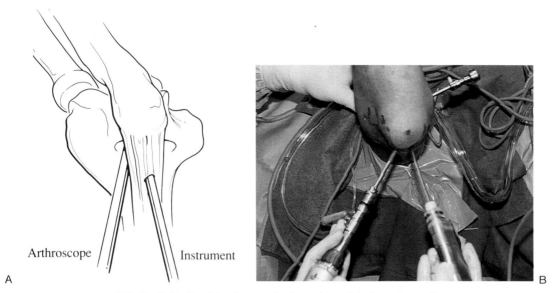

Arthroscope

Instrument

A

B

FIG. 7. A, B: Combined posterior lateral–straight lateral portals.

synovial villi that become fibrotic and are then detached and float free within the elbow joint (12).

Loose bodies within the elbow joint are of concern for several reasons. First of all, they may cause mechanical symptoms such as catching or locking of the elbow joint with motion. They may also cause wear and destruction of the chondral surfaces if they become caught between these surfaces.

Loose bodies may be found in many locations within the elbow joint. Because many of these loose bodies are the result of osteochondritic lesions of the capitellum or osteochondral fractures from lateral compression injuries, loose bodies will often be found in the posterior and posterolateral compartments of the elbow. However, it is not uncommon for these loose bodies to migrate within the elbow joint and to be found in the anterior compartment as well (Fig. 8).

Surgical Approach

The arthroscopic surgical approach for removal of loose bodies consists of a thorough and meticulous evaluation of the whole joint. The joint is sequentially examined through the anterolateral, anteromedial, lateral, and posterolateral portals. Loose bodies may often be encapsulated or densely adherent to surrounding soft tissue. It is necessary to use a full-radius resector to release these soft tissue attachments so that the loose body may be grasped and removed from the joint. Loose bodies within the elbow joint are commonly large and may require an extension of the capsular puncture for removal. If a large loose body is encountered in the anterior compartment of the elbow prior to evaluation of the lateral and posterior compartments of the elbow, it should be left in place until the entire elbow joint has been exam-

ined. In this way, an extension of the capsular incision anteriorly is not performed prior to the complete evaluation of the entire elbow joint, preventing extensive extravasation of arthroscopic fluid from the anterior capsular rent into the surrounding soft tissues and reducing the risk of potential neurovascular compromise. If an extension of an arthroscopic portal is required for loose body removal, the portal may simply be closed with a single suture.

Osteochondrosis of the Capitellum

The elbow is subject to a variety of injuries, which are the result of biomechanical stresses during throwing and

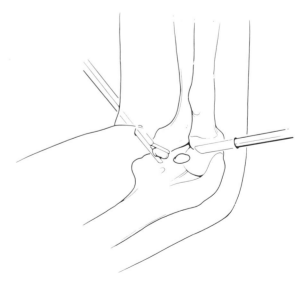

FIG. 8. Removal of loose bodies.

similar motions. When throwing, the elbow is subjected to a valgus moment as the hand, forearm, and ball lag behind the trunk and upper arm during the acceleration phase of throwing. This valgus moment results in tension injuries to the medial capsuloligamentous structures and lateral compression injuries to the bony structures (9).

Although in the past Panner's disease and osteochondritis dissecans were felt to be separate entities, it has now become apparent that these are different stages of the same disease process. The basic pathologic process producing this disease entity has been well described. The valgus stress imposed on the elbow during throwing results in lateral compression injuries to the lateral bony structures of the capitellum and radial head. Repetitive microtrauma results in repeated insults to the vulnerable blood supply of the humeral capitellum and in vascular insufficiency to the capitellum, with subsequent alteration of enchondral ossification. The end result of this sequence of events depends on the age of the patient, the type and level of patient activities, and the severity of the original lesion (8).

The term "Panner's disease" is most often applied to patients in the early spectrum of this disease, from 5 to 10 years of age. These patients experience a fragmentation of the entire ossific nucleus of the capitellum, which tends to totally reconstitute with conservative treatment and does not result in destruction of the capitellum or the production of loose bodies. The term "osteochondritis dissecans" is used for patients in the older spectrum of this disease. These patients exhibit partial involvement of the capitellum, with frequent fragmentation of the involved area. These fragments may become separated from their bed and form loose bodies within the elbow joint (7). The patients in this group tend to have the worst prognosis for a good result with conservative therapy, and may require arthroscopic surgery. The indications for surgery for osteochondrosis of the humeral capitellum include a locked elbow, intraarticular loose bodies, or the failure of conservative treatment over an extended period of time to control pain.

Surgical Approach

The arthroscopic surgical approach for an osteochondritic lesion of the humeral capitellum includes both a thorough inspection of the lesion of the capitellum and a complete evaluation of the entire elbow joint to search for possible loose bodies.

The osteochondritic defect of the capitellum can be best visualized through the straight lateral portal (Fig. 9). Instruments are introduced through a second straight lateral portal. Through this portal the lesion of the capitellum may be palpated and its entire extent defined. After the entire extent of the lesion is identified the fragmented portion of the lesion may be elevated with a small osteotome and removed with a Schlessinger clamp. Following removal of the large fragmented pieces, the base of the lesion is debrided using a curette and a high-speed motorized bur. The base of the lesion is debrided down to healthy bleeding bone. In our experience, simple excision of the fragmented portion of the capitellum and curettage of the base of the lesion to healthy bleeding bone gives the most satisfactory result. We do not recommend pinning back a fragmented piece of the capitellum or drilling the base of the lesion to obtain bleeding. Following complete removal of the fragmented portion of the capitellum, the remainder of the elbow joint is thoroughly inspected to ensure that no loose bodies are present in the anterior or posterior aspect of the elbow.

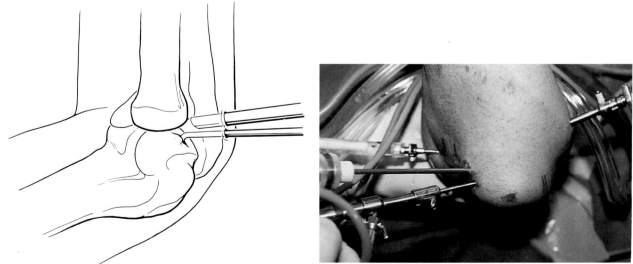

A   B

FIG. 9. A, B: Debridement of osteochondritis dissecans capitellum.

Arthroscopic reduction and screw fixation of the osteochondritic defect in an attempt to promote healing of the defect has been described (7). However, this is technically a very demanding procedure and long-term results of this technique are not known.

Synovial Diseases

Systemic inflammatory diseases such as rheumatoid arthritis often affect the elbow joint. These inflammatory arthritides produce both mechanical and biochemical problems within the elbow joint. Mechanically, the expansive synovitis associated with rheumatoid arthritis can stretch the capsuloligamentous structures about the joint. As these capsuloligamentous structures are progressively stretched over a prolonged period of time, the joint loses its ligamentous integrity. With the loss of ligamentous integrity about the elbow, the biomechanics of the joint articulations are altered, and areas of uneven wear and force distribution are produced, resulting in erosion and destruction of the joint articular surfaces. Biomechanically, rheumatoid arthritis is associated with antigen/antibody deposition within the tissues, followed by migration of phagocytic and lymphocytic cells into the joint. These cells release collagenases and proteinases that destroy the cartilaginous network of the articular surfaces (6).

The goal of synovectomy in rheumatoid arthritis and other inflammatory arthritides is to remove synovial tissue within the joint that causes expansive synovitis leading to mechanical destruction of the joint and the deposition of antigen/antibody complexes that initiate the biochemical destruction of the articular surfaces.

The technique of arthroscopic synovectomy of the elbow joint requires utilization of all the standard arthroscopic portals for elbow joint arthroscopy. In this way the entire joint may be thoroughly evaluated and a complete synovectomy performed using a full-radius resector. The capsuloligamentous and musculotendinous units spanning the elbow joint are not disturbed by an incision with an arthroscopic synovectomy, and an early aggressive range of motion and physical therapy program may be initiated.

Osteophyte Formation on the Olecranon

In addition to medial tension injuries and lateral compression injuries, the posterior aspect of the elbow is subjected to degenerative changes of the olecranon and the olecranon fossa during the act of throwing. These degenerative changes are the result of two mechanisms: (a) forced hyperextension of the olecranon into the olecranon fossa, and (b) shear forces between the olecranon and the olecranon fossa secondary to the valgus moment placed on the elbow during throwing. The combination

of these forces leads to the formation of posterior and posteromedial osteophytes of the olecranon and chondromalacia of the olecranon fossa (Fig. 10). The combination of these two mechanisms has been termed the *valgus extension overload syndrome* and is most commonly seen in high-caliber throwing athletes such as baseball pitchers (4). The degenerative changes and osteophytic spurring that occur may result in decreased motion of the elbow and pain, which limits performance.

The initial results of excision of posterior osteophytes in such cases were disappointing, and some authors felt that the return to competitive pitching would seldom occur (13). However, as this overuse syndrome has become better defined, the results of excision of the osteophytes, with return to competitive pitching, have become more promising and continue to improve with the advent of arthroscopic techniques for excision of such osteophytes (10).

The pathology in the valgus extension overload syndrome can best be evaluated through a posterolateral portal. When this portal has been established, a straight posterior portal can be established under direct visualization for introduction of the arthroscopic surgical equipment. Initially all the soft tissue and synovitis of the posterior compartment is resected with a full-radius resector so that the entire bony margins of the osteophytes can be readily visualized. At this point an osteotome can be brought in through the straight posterior portal, and the osteophytes of the posterior and posteromedial corner of the olecranon may be removed (Fig. 11). Next, a high-speed bur may be brought in through the straight posterior portal, and the remainder of the resection of the posterior and posteromedial osteophytes may be accomplished with the bur. At this point, a full-radius resector is reintroduced through the straight posterior portal, the margins of the olecranon are debrided

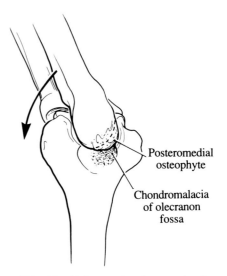

FIG. 10. Valgus extension overload.

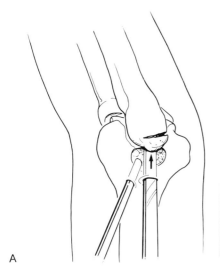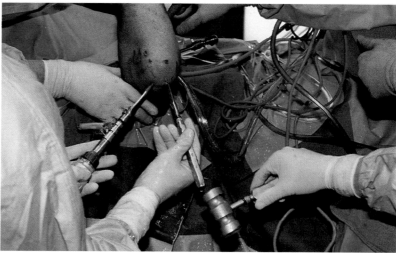

FIG. 11. A, B: Osteophytic removal of valgus extension overload.

to a smooth surface, and the areas of chondromalacia within the olecranon fossa are also debrided to a smooth surface. Under direct visualization, the elbow may then be put through a full range of motion to ensure that any impinging posterior osteophytes have been resected.

Posttraumatic and Postsurgical Adhesions

Posttraumatic and postsurgical adhesions are dreaded complications following trauma to the elbow, as well as open surgical procedures about the elbow joint. The elbow is often immobilized in 90° of flexion after such injuries. In this position, fibrous adhesions may form in the anterior capsular region of the elbow and span the anterior aspect of the joint, causing a significant loss of extension.

Anterior capsular adhesions are most readily evaluated through both anterolateral and anteromedial portals. Utilization of both of these portals allows a full inspection of the entire anterior compartment of the elbow as well as the anterior capsule. The fibrous adhesions can then be fully resected using a full-radius resector. Following complete release of the adhesions in the anterior aspect of the elbow, the joint may be manipulated into extension. After the anterior capsular adhesions have been excised, a thorough inspection of the posterior aspect of the elbow must be performed to ensure that there is no residual mechanical block to extension in the posterior aspect of the elbow.

The success of arthroscopic release of adhesions in the elbow to regain range of motion is dependent on an early aggressive physical therapy program. This may include stretching casts, dynasplints, and orthotic devices that aid the patient in maintaining extension postoperatively.

COMPLICATIONS

As with any arthroscopic surgical procedure, potential complications do exist. Although septic arthritis is a very rare complication following arthroscopy of the elbow, it does occur. With proper sterilization of the arthroscopic equipment and with meticulous attention to sterile technique, the rate of incidence should be no higher than that expected for shoulder and knee arthroscopy.

Neurovascular injury is probably the most common potential complication of elbow arthroscopy because of the close proximity of the major neurovascular structures to the arthroscopic portals (5,11). Meticulous attention to the anatomic details and technical considerations of elbow arthroscopy that have been well described will prevent direct injury to the neurovascular structures of the elbow.

Neurovascular compromise may also result from extravasation of fluid into the soft tissues about the elbow. If extravasation is excessive, an actual compartment syndrome in the forearm could develop. Therefore, particular attention must be paid to swelling about the elbow through the entire operative procedure. Technically, it is important to establish portals at the first attempt and to maintain that placement throughout the entire procedure. When moving from the anterior to the posterior portal, it is important to leave the cannulas in place anteriorly so that the rent in the capsule is sealed off by the cannula. If the cannulas are removed, extravasation of fluid through the anterior portals into the surrounding soft tissue may occur, and potential neurovascular compromise is possible. The surgeon must constantly watch the degree of swelling and be prepared to stop the procedure if indicated.

CONCLUSIONS

The ability to treat intraarticular pathology of the elbow arthroscopically continues to increase as arthroscopic instrumentation and technical skills improve. Advantages of arthroscopic treatment of elbow pathology include: (a) a more thorough visualization of the entire elbow joint; (b) a decrease in postoperative scarring; (c) the ability to initiate a more aggressive and earlier postoperative physical therapy program; (d) a decreased change of intraarticular infection. At the same time, arthroscopy of the elbow is a technically demanding procedure that requires a thorough understanding of the anatomy of the elbow as it applies to portal placement and the relationships of intraarticular structures. It also requires a thorough understanding of basic arthroscopic surgical techniques that can then be modified as necessary for application to the elbow.

With a thorough understanding of these anatomical and technical considerations, elbow arthroscopy can offer a significant advance and improvement in treatment of intraarticular pathology of the elbow.

REFERENCES

1. Andrews JR, et al. Arthroscopy of the elbow. *Clin Sports Med* 1986;5:653–662.
2. Andrews JR, Angelo RL. Elbow arthroscopy. In: Wadsworth TG, ed. *The Elbow.* 2nd Ed. New York: Churchill Livingstone, 1988.
3. Carson WG, Andrews JR. Arthroscopy of the elbow. *Arthroscopy* 1985;1:97–107.
4. DeHaven KE, Evarts CM. Throwing injuries of the elbow in athletes. *Orthop Clin North Am* 1973;4:301–308.
5. Guhl JF. Arthroscopy and arthroscopic surgery of the elbow. *Orthopedics* 1985;8:1290–1296.
6. Indelicato PA. Correctable elbow lesions in professional baseball players: A review of 25 cases. *Am J Sports Med* 1979;7:72–75.
7. Johnson LJ. Elbow arthroscopy. In: *Arthroscopy Surgery, Principles and Practice.* St. Louis: CV Mosby, 1986, pp. 1446–1477.
8. Singer KM. Osteochondrosis of the humeral capitellum. *Am J Sports Med* 1984;12:351.
9. Slocum DB. Classification of the elbow injuries from baseball pitching. *Texas Med* 1968;64:48–53.
10. Small NC. Complications in arthroscopy: the knee and other joints. *Arthroscopy* 1986;2:253–258.
11. Thomas MA. Radial nerve damage as a complication of elbow arthroscopy. *Clin Orthop* 1987;215:130–131.
12. Turek SL. The elbow. In: *Orthopaedics: Principles and Their Application.* Philadelphia: JB Lippincott, 1984, pp. 967–984.
13. Wilson FD, Andrews JR. Valgus extension overload in the pitching elbow. *Am J Sports Med* 1983;2:83.

SUBJECT INDEX

Subject Index

Radial collateral elbow ligament, 137, 140–141
Radial collateral wrist ligament, 10
Radial head (elbow)
　anatomy, 137–138, 141, 143, 145
　　pediatric patients, 146
　anteromedial portal view, 167
　dislocations, 151
　excision, 135–136
　fracture, 147–149
　and landmark identification, 160, 162
　posterolateral portal view, 133
　proximal medial portal view, 134
　straight lateral portal view, 169
　surgical approach, 172
Radial head-capitellum radiography, 143, 145
Radial midcarpal portal, 6–7, 13–14, 66, 68, 78–80
Radial neck fractures, 148–149
Radial nerve (elbow)
　anatomy, 163–165
　iatrogenic injury, 170
Radial nerve (wrist)
　anatomy, 6
　iatrogenic injury, 124
Radial notch, 137, 140–141
Radial tubercle, 137–138
Radiocapitellar joint, 133
Radiocarpal joint
　arthrography, 26–27, 29–30
　and scapholunate tear treatment, 78–80
Radiolunate ligament, 7–9
Radiolunotriquetral ligament
　arthroscopic anatomy, 7–9
　surgical technique, 63, 65
Radionuclide imaging, 25–26, 28–29, 32
Radioscaphocapitate ligament
　arthroscopic anatomy, 7–10, 14
　surgical technique, 63, 65
Radioscaphoid angle, 20, 22–23
Radioscapholunate ligament, 7–10, 12
Radiotriquetral ligament, 14
Radioulnar joint (elbow). *See also* Distal radioulnar wrist joint
　posterolateral view, 133
　straight lateral portal view, 169
Radioulnar ligaments, 12, 85, 87–89
Radioulnar subluxation, 46–48
Radius (elbow), 132, 139, 147
Radius (wrist)
　arthroscopic anatomy, 12, 15
　carpal relationships, 40, 43
　plain-film radiography, 20, 22
Recurrent radial artery, 165
Reflex sympathetic dystrophy, 26, 29, 124–125
Rheumatoid arthritis, 117–120, 177
Ronguers, 58

Rotatory scaphoid subluxation, 20–21
Rotatory subluxation of the navicular, 41, 44

S
Salter-Harris injuries, 150
Scaphoid bone
　arthroscopic examination, 66, 68
　fractures, 28, 32, 34–36
　plain-film radiography, 19–21, 24
　signet ring appearance, 20–21
Scaphoid facet of the radius, 65–66
Scaphoid fat stripe, 19
Scaphoid fossa, 10
Scaphoid fracture
　avascular necrosis, 34–36
　imaging, 28, 32, 34–36
　radionuclide imaging, 28
Scaphoid ligament, 7–8
Scapholunate angle
　and carpal instability, 42
　normal appearance, 40
　plain-film radiography, 20, 22–23, 40
Scapholunate articulation, 14
Scapholunate dissociation
　imaging, 19–20, 41, 44, 74–75, 78
　physical examination, 74
Scapholunate joint
　arthroscopic examination, 66, 69
　pinning of, 79–80
Scapholunate ligament
　arthroscopic anatomy, 63, 65–66
　arthroscopic examination, 63, 65–66
　histology, 76–77, 80
Scapholunate ligament tear
　arthrography, 30
　imaging, 41, 44, 78–79
　treatment, 78–80
Scaphotrapeziotrapezoid articulation, 15
Scaphotrapeziotrapezoid joint, 66, 69
Scaphotrapeziotrapezoid portal, 6–7, 15, 66, 68
Scleroderma, 117
Scrub nurse, 56
Semilunar notch, 137
Semisupinated wrist radiography, 25, 27
Septic arthritis
　elbow, 155, 178
　wrist, 119
"Shuck" test, 74
Sigmoid notch, 15, 88, 90
"Signet ring" sign, 20–21, 41, 74–75
"Soft spot," 174
"Spike" fracture, 101–102, 104
"Split fracture," 101
Sporotrichosis, 119
Spur formation, 154–156
Stabilization devices, 60
Stellate axillary block, 125

Steroid-dependent arthritis patients, 119
Straight lateral elbow portal, 168–169, 173–174
Straight posterior elbow portal, 168–169, 174–175
Superficial radial nerve
　elbow, 163–165
　wrist, 124
Supination scan, 47
Supracondylar fractures, 149–150
Surgical assistant, 56–57
Surgical technique
　elbow arthroscopy, 160–169, 171–179
　wrist arthroscopy, 63–71
Surgical team, 56–57, 161
Suspension devices, 60–61
Sympathetic ganglion block, 125
Synovectomy
　elbow, 135, 177
　wrist, 119–120
Synovial chondromatosis, 155–156
Synovial tuft, 8, 10, 63, 65
Synovitis
　elbow, 177
　wrist, 91, 119–120
Systemic lupus erythematosus, 117

T
Tendinitis, 154
"Tennis elbow," 153–154
Tomography
　elbow examination, 146
　wrist examination, 25, 28
Toughy 20-gauge needle, 93–94
Tourniquet control, 160
Traction tower, 55–56, 61, 63–64, 104
Trans-scaphoid volar perilunate dislocation, 39–40
Transient nerve palsies, 170
Trapezium, 25, 27
Triangular fibrocartilage. *See also* Triangular fibrocartilage complex
　anatomy, 7–8, 11–16
　arthroscopic examination, 65, 67
　and distal radioulnar joint stabilization, 98–100
　rheumatoid arthritis, 120
　traumatic lesions, 88–90
Triangular fibrocartilage articular disc, 97
Triangular fibrocartilage complex, 85–96
　anatomy, 12, 85–89
　arthrography, tears, 30, 49
　arthroscopic examination, 90–96
　diagnostic arthroscopy, 90–96
　and distal forearm fracture, 105, 108
　histologic section, 86